Managing and Preventing Prostate Disorders

THE NATURAL ALTERNATIVES

Managing and Preventing Prostate Disorders

THE NATURAL ALTERNATIVES

George L. Redmon, Ph.D., N.D.

HOHM PRESS

Cover design: Kim Johansen
Layout and design: J. Pratt, Alpha-Cat Design

Library of Congress Cataloging in Publication Data:
Redmon, George L., 1952-
    Managing and preventing prostate disorders: the natural alternatives /
    George L. Redmon
    p.cm.
    Includes bibliographical references and index.
    ISBN 0-934252-97-1 (alk. paper)
    1. Prostate—Diseases—Alternative treatment. 2. Prostate—Cancer—
    Alternative treatment. I. Title

RC899 .R35 2000
 616.6'5—dc21

                            99-045214

Disclaimer: It is not the intent of the author to diagnose or prescribe. Nor is it the purpose of this book to replace the services of your physician. The material is intended for educational purposes only. It is advisable to consult a doctor for any condition that may require his or her services.

HOHM PRESS
P.O. Box 2501
Prescott, AZ 86302
800-381-2700
Printed in the U.S.A. on recycled paper using soy ink.
http://www.hohmpress.com

This book is dedicated to the memory of Carlton Fredericks, Ph.D. (1910–1987), a pioneer of nutritional pharmacology. His efforts and commitment, as well as those of others, to bringing alternative health methods to the forefront, have encouraged prevention versus treatment—a view now poised to become the primary focus of managed healthcare in the twenty-first century. His work has shaped and molded my thought and my battles to escape the etiological progression of disease.

When nutritional treatment helps the suffering, my joy is tinged with a note of regret, for such victories are often monuments to lost opportunities for prevention.

—*Carlton Fredericks, Ph.D.*

ACKNOWLEDGMENTS

I would like to express sincere gratitude and appreciation to Eric C. Dettrey and his secretarial staff, especially Lorri Giebel, for the exceptional editorial and copy work done on this manuscript.

This author is also greatly indebted to the countless pioneers whose insights and intestinal fortitude gave birth to the notion that there may be a better and more natural way to correct the metabolic capacity of human physiological systems under distress. Their efforts have helped to dispel the notion that the restoration of human metabolic pathways and maintaining a healthy internal environment were the same as pharmaceutical intervention.

Gratitude goes to my editor, Regina Sara Ryan of Hohm Press, for guidance and the uncanny ability to elicit attention to detail, thus fostering critical thinking. Her work has had a profound impact on me as a researcher.

The author owes a sincere debt of gratitude to Ms. Andrea Foster, director of the Holistic Resource and Referral Network of Houston, Texas, for her emotional and professional support in the completion of this manuscript.

Lastly, I thank my wife Brenda and my family for their undying support of my efforts in the completion of this project.

CONTENTS

We know that there is no scientific proof that any of the prostate surgeries or treatments do extend a man's life. If the same man opts for "watchful waiting," he would probably live another sixteen years without the discomfort, risk, or complication of surgery.

—*Arnold Fox, M.D.*

What is considered appropriate treatment is to wait until the problem is severe enough to need surgery. There are situations where a disease can progress while you're not aware of it, but with "BPH" (Benign Prostatic Hyperplasia) the disease is the symptom, basically. The disease is the growth of the prostate, but the symptom is blockage of the urinary tract.

—*Michael Janson, M.D.*

Here's the bottom line. Before submitting to surgery for an enlarged prostate, ask whether it's safe to wait, then do so. If something must be done, consider first one of the non-surgical alternatives already available.

—*Isadore Rosenfeld, M.D.*

I knew that most of the men who I was operating on for prostate problems would probably never have sex again. I just couldn't do it anymore. I knew there must be a better way.

—*James Balch, M.D.*

PREFACE

The comments of the prominent physicians just quoted imply
that the best treatment for prostate problems may be to keep a
watchful eye on the progression of the symptoms and/or the
diagnosed presence of cancer. Their opinions also suggest that
there can be serious risk, discomfort, and quality-of-life issues
associated with surgical intervention. Finally, their remarks propose that the use of an existing, alternative, non-surgical approach should be given strong consideration in the treatment
of prostate disturbances.

The key question here is would these alternative options
apply to the benign (non-cancerous) symptoms from BPH, short
for benign prostatic hyperplasia (an enlargement of the prostate
gland), prostatitis (inflammation of the prostate gland), or the
evidence of cancer of the prostate gland? According to these
doctors, watchful waiting would be a viable option in all of the
aforementioned cases.

Watchful waiting must be distinguished from "plain old waiting," procrastinating or stalling. During the period of watchful
waiting, various protocols or alternative, non-surgical treatment options are explored and administered. We will cover
many of these options throughout this book. This approach is
in total contrast to simply doing nothing. Based on the severity
or non-severity of the prostate disturbance, non-surgical intervention is the cornerstone of watchful waiting.

In his book *The Best Treatment,* Dr. Isadore Rosenfeld asks
us to remember the days when doctors recommended that any

child whose tonsils were enlarged be scheduled for a tonsil-lectomy. This procedure is rarely done today, but the same restraint does not yet apply to an enlarged prostate. Fortunately, according to Rosenfeld, "medical thinking is moving in that direction." In fact, he predicts that in the not-too-distant future, prostatectomy (removal of the entire prostate) will become a procedure of the past.

In the meantime, while many health care professionals today insist that watchful waiting may be a much more viable option, which modality or combination of approaches to use in this waiting game is the important question.

It is my hope that *Managing and Preventing Prostate Disorders* will help make finding the answer to that question a little less difficult.

WHY "SIMPLY WAITING" IS NOT AN OPTION

Problems associated with prostate disturbances are not to be taken lightly. In fact, current data indicate that one out of every ten men in the United States will develop prostate cancer in his lifetime. Additionally, as noted by Patrick C. Walsh, M.D., Director of the Department of Urology at the Johns Hopkins University School of Medicine, few men who live a normal life span (about seventy-four years) will be fortunate enough to be spared some difficulties arising from prostate disorders.

While current statistics show white males have a one in eleven chance of developing prostate cancer, the odds are worse—one in seven—if you are an African-American male. According to the American Cancer Society, some 200,000 new cases of prostate cancer are diagnosed each year. Over 30,000 men die of this disease every year—one every thirteen minutes. In fact, prostate cancer is the second most prevalent kind of cancer in men, second only to skin cancer, and is much more prevalent than breast cancer is in women (although not as highly publicized). In fact, the incidence of prostate cancer is thirty-three percent higher than the incidence of breast cancer. Paradoxically, of the ten leading causes of death in this country, American males lead in eight of them.

The probability that an individual male in this culture will develop some sort of prostate dysfunction is high. So high, researchers estimate, that if you are a male over forty and haven't experienced some sort of prostate dysfunction, the probability of that happening is two to one by the time you reach fifty-nine.

You don't have to be on the wrong side of these statistics, however. Dr. Elliot J. Howard, a medical internist at the Lenox Hill Hospital in New York City and author of *Health Risk,* maintains that you have the opportunity to take control over many of the risk factors associated with many of today's degenerative diseases. He adamantly contends that you can take steps right now to help you live a long, vigorous life, staying healthy and active well into your eighties and even nineties.

I strongly agree with Dr. Howard's assessment, as I am a former cancer patient, having battled and won over twenty years ago. It was 1974 when I found out I had cancer. That year also changed my life, and actually gave me the insight to realize that health did not exist in a vacuum. My journey back to health has become a lifelong adventure. I have come to realize that the key to maintaining radiant health begins and ends with me.

Please do not be discouraged if you are in ill health right now. This present setback should be viewed as an opportunity to devise and implement a total wellness program to restore and maintain optimal health. Julian Whitaker, M.D., one of America's most notable medical doctors, incorporates the use of well-documented alternative medical modalities into his private practice and advocates a total wellness program to help you regain health, as well as to prevent disease. This same sentiment is also expressed by Harry G. Preuss, M.D., and Brenda Adderly, M.H.A., authors of *Prostate Cure.* These researchers maintain that your best weapon against prostate disturbances is to "live well."

THE PURPOSE OF THIS BOOK

My intention is to give you an overview of some options you may not be fully aware of. The overall goal of this book is to help you establish a lifelong preventive plan that is geared toward maintaining good prostate health, as well as overall health. However, you will note that many of the alternative protocols, products and nutritional regimens outlined here can also be used to fight cancer of the prostate. In considering any options mentioned, therefore, thorough discussion with your healthcare professional is necessary and recommended.

The following quote by Dr. Whitaker puts the goal of the book into proper perspective:

> From a doctor's standpoint, preventive medicine can be somewhat boring. From your perspective, however, preventive medicine is likely to be the most valuable insurance policy you will ever have. Many of your friends and family will unfortunately succumb to degenerative disease and "go under the knife" while you will, hopefully, be watching on the sidelines in a state of good health. (p. 27)

INTRODUCTION

Over twelve million men in the U.S. suffer from some sort of prostate dysfunction, and about one-half of these men require some form of treatment. It is predicted that by the year 2020 this number will double. Why has the incidence of prostate disorder skyrocketed over the last four or five decades? Many researchers claim that this rising trend is a direct result of an aging population living longer. This argument, however, is disputed by many alternative as well as conventional researchers. While there is a direct correlation with aging and an increased incidence of benign prostatic hyperplasia, aging in and of itself is only one part of this degenerative puzzle.

Deepak Chopra, M.D., suggests that although there are certain biological clocks predetermined within us that will cause some change in organs or bodily functions, ninety-nine percent of our vitality, health and healing capabilities remain stable and theoretically sound throughout life. Deepak Chopra, Richard Passwater, Ph.D., Michael Murray, N.D., Joseph Pizzorno, N.D., Andrew Weil, M.D., and countless other researchers and doctors maintain that the passing of time is not the culprit in the diseases usually associated with aging. Rather, negative features associated with "aging" are more often the result of derangement of the body's metabolic machinery caused by unhealthy lifestyles, improper diet, increased drug and alcohol consumption, stress, environmental changes, oxidative stress, and a host of other factors.

Dr. James Balch, a nationally-known urologist and author of the highly acclaimed *Prescription for Nutritional Healing,* has stated that there may be better approaches to dealing with prostate disorders than the current medical model of drugs and surgery. Balch and others note that while prostate disorders are also prevalent in other countries, many of our European and Asian counterparts suffer far less from this malady.

The key question here is *why?* Why are doctors abroad less likely to prescribe drugs and surgery, preferring the use of natural medicines to attack prostate disorders? Why do over ninety percent of the physicians in Germany disregard the types of drugs used in the United States to treat prostate disturbances? What natural remedies are they using and why are they so successful with them? A more important question in this insidious paradox is, *Why aren't we utilizing these treatments and conducting research into their efficiency?*

In the U.S., the answer is enmeshed in the political battle to remain a one-dimensional health care system in which treatment prevails over prevention. According to a 1993 survey by the World Health Organization (*Alternative Medicine Digest* 16, pp. 82–83), this closed approach to health care is a major reason why the U.S. is ranked eighteenth in overall health, despite its wealth and size. The World Health Organization maintains that in many smaller countries, such as Sweden, where a "pluralistic" approach to health care exists—meaning an open society where both conventional and alternative modalities are openly accepted and practiced—the state of overall health outpaces that in the U.S.

AN ALTERNATIVE MOVEMENT

The past trend of dismissing non-invasive alternative treatment is changing, however. Dr. David Eisenberg from the Harvard School of Medicine reported in 1993 that 33.8 percent of Americans had used some form of alternative therapy in 1990. In a recent follow-up study (1998), Dr. Eisenberg revealed that the use of alternative therapies (now being called "complementary") increased from 33.8 percent in 1990 to a whopping 42.1 percent in 1997.

Because the number of men around the globe who suffer from benign prostatic hyperplasia is increasing, questions concerning the efficacy of many non-surgical procedures, as well as non-drug-related supplements, are also being raised.

THE PROBLEM WITH BPH

Benign prostatic hyperplasia is characterized by some generally annoying symptoms—urinary frequency, especially at night; pain with ejaculation; incomplete urination (starting and stopping, dribbling), and incontinence (loss of bladder control). The negative ramifications of these symptoms will be covered in detail in Chapters One and Two.

These symptoms are warning signals that need to be investigated and evaluated by a qualified medical professional. You cannot diagnose the severity of BPH and its related compilations for yourself. Some symptoms of BPH may simply indicate the need to make a few adjustments in diet and lifestyle. However, since this disorder can be deadly, medical assessment is recommended and should be sought. According to Carlton Fredericks, Ph.D.,

> Since prostate cancer is to men what breast cancer is to women, it is vitally important that men with symptoms of prostate enlargement (BPH) undergo a thorough examination to be sure that it is benign (non-cancerous) rather than malignant. (p. 156)

Whatever verdict follows the assessment, recognize that a lot has changed over the last twenty years. Numerous options, both surgical and non-invasive, should be discussed with your personal physician, your family, and knowledgeable friends.

To assess the overall ramifications of these emerging options, this book is organized as follows:

Part One—The Nature of the Prostate Gland, includes:
Chapter 1. The Anatomy of a Prostate Gland
Chapter 2. Understanding Prostate Disturbances
Chapter 3. Diagnosing Prostate Disturbances

The overall goal of the first three chapters is to give an overview of the prostate gland—its function, general anatomy, location in the body, biological need, and associated problems.

Part Two—The Treatment Options, covers:

Chapter 4. Conventional Treatments
Chapter 5. Alternative Treatments

Here you will find a general overview of many standard medical procedures, as well as some past and present alternative modalities. This section will also consider some of the emerging protocols used outside of the United States that have proven to be successful in treating prostate disturbances.

Part Three—Preventive Measures, covers:

Chapter 6. Natural Born Medicaments
Chapter 7. Proper Nutrition As Preventive Medicine

These two chapters will introduce you to some of the most popular and widely used supplements that have been shown to be as effective as many of their drug counterparts in the treatment of BPH, without the negative side effects. How an individual could be contributing to, accelerating and/or possibly causing the development of his prostate discomfort via improper dietary habits is discussed here.

Part Four—Managing Prostate Health, includes:

Chapter 8. Designing a Personal Maintenance Plan
Chapter 9. Getting the Help You Need—plus The Holistic Health Directory

In this section you will learn how to set up a plan that is designed to promote lifelong prostate health. This segment will also give you a variety of options and contacts, both conventional and alternative, to assist you or your loved ones in finding the appropriate help.

PART ONE

The Nature of the Prostate Gland

The human body is not like the "Wonderful One-Hoss Shay" of Oliver Wendell Holmes. It is not fixed in structure and function. It does not age all together.

—*Michael Colgan, Ph.D., CCN*

CHAPTER ONE

THE ANATOMY OF
A PROSTATE GLAND

This chapter will address the following vital questions:

- Where is the prostate gland located in the body?
- What is its function?
- What other organs does the prostate interact with?
- How is this gland linked to sexual function?
- Why should men give careful attention to this gland?
- What are the complications associated with prostate dysfunction?

According to Barry King, Ph.D., and Mary Jane Showers, R.N., Ph.D., in *Human Anatomy and Physiology:* "The prostate gland lies beneath the bladder and surrounds the first portion of the urethra. Around the urethra the smooth muscle fibers form a ring that is called the internal sphincter of the bladder. The ducts of the gland open into the urethra." (p. 399)

The prostate gland is a male sex organ. Red-brown in color, about the size of an English walnut, this little gland does some unique things. Every male should learn how to take care of it, for it is intimately involved with sexual gratification and can have a profound effect on emotional, physiological and biological aspects of overall health. The prostate gland should be given the same lifelong attention and intense concern by men as women give "breast health."

PROSTATE 101

In a mature male, the prostate gland weighs only about seven-tenths of an ounce. At birth it is about the size of a pea. By puberty it will increase to the size of an almond. Because of the natural increase of sex hormone activity during adolescence, the prostate gland will accelerate in growth. By the time a man reaches age twenty or thirty, the prostate gland has reached the size of a walnut or chestnut.

The prostate gland resides just below the bladder. It can be found in the lower part of the abdomen at the base of or in back of the penis. If a man were able to look inside himself, the prostate gland would appear as a little spot just beneath the urinary bladder, directly in front of the rectum. (See Figure 1.1.)

Notice the connection of the prostate and the urethra. The prostate gland actually wraps around the urethra, the narrow portal that runs through the penis. Once urine is expelled from the bladder it is transported through the urethra, and then exits the body. This is also the way your ejaculate travels, through the urethra, before being expelled at the moment of heightened sexual stimulation.

If you could take a trip in a small vessel down into the deep recesses of the prostate, as in many organs of the body, you would find a network of many glands and ducts. In fact, the prostate gland is an aggregate of about forty tubuloaveolar (tubes with air sacs) glands, which are separated from each other by smooth muscle tissue, as well as by dense fibrous tissue. Through this network the prostate gland releases a thin alkaline fluid known as "prostatic secretion," which combines with sperm when a man ejaculates. This fluid passes through the network of ducts, and when it combines with sperm,

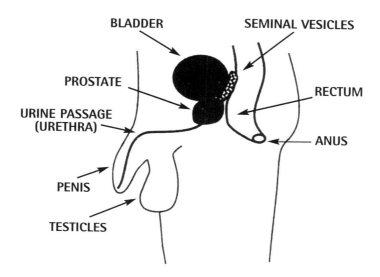

Figure 1.1 Source: Wallner, K., M.D., *Prostate Cancer: A Non-Surgical Perspective.* Canaan, New York: Smart Medicine Press, 1996, p. 7. Used with permission.

semen is formed. Prostatic fluid makes up a large percentage of semen. As a point of reference, semen actually consists of only about five percent sperm. The majority of the semen is produced by the seminal vesicles and the prostate gland.

The muscles that surround the prostate actually contract with orgasm. They are responsible for facilitating the movement of the mixture of sperm and fluids through the urethra during ejaculation.

THE MIRACULOUS FUNCTIONS OF THE PROSTATE

One could argue that without the miraculous feats of the prostate gland the continuation of the human race would be in jeopardy. During sexual intercourse, when the muscles of the prostate gland contract, causing its fluids to be released into the urethral tract, some important biological functions occur. This fluid has a number of vital responsibilities such as:

1. Protecting sperm cells from the acidic environment of the vagina.
2. Providing nourishment to sperm cells.
3. Promoting prostaglandin production (hormone-like fatty acids), which stimulates the cervix to widen, thereby allowing sperm to pass through the uterus, encouraging fertilization.
4. Protecting the urinary tract from harmful substances or toxins.

Obviously, the prostate gland should be cared for, meaning that every man should have in place, early in life—from the mid-twenties to early thirties—a lifelong plan that is geared toward preventing prostate disturbances.

THE INVISIBLE HAND OF NATURE

Natural enlargement of the prostate happens as cells inside the gland begin to multiply a little more rapidly. By the time you reach your forty-fifth birthday and into your later years, this sudden cell proliferation causes the prostate to enlarge, sometimes as much as ten times its normal size. When this happens, the prostate gland will begin to tighten the normal hold it has on the urethra.

Visualize placing a straw in your open hand, then clenching your fist around it—first loosely, then very tightly. This is an example of what an enlarged prostate gland is doing to your urethra. And this mishap can spell big trouble. The location of the prostate is a concern. The enlargement can cause the normal flow of urine to become obstructed, with grave consequences. Early warning signs that the prostate is pinching or clamping down too tightly around the urethra range from frequent urination, increased urgency to urinate, and stop-and-go flow of urine during urination, to pain in the pelvic or rectal areas. Lower back pain, pain in the testicles, nausea, dizziness, and unexplained tendency toward sleeping may also be signs of impending prostate disturbances. An enlarged prostate gland that is obstructing the normal flow of urine from the body can lead to kidney and bladder dysfunction. According to Richard E. Berger, M.D., Director of Reproduction and Sexual Medicine at the University of Washington Medical Center in Seattle, kidney dysfunction has a tendency to make you want to sleep more. (Editors of *Prevention Magazine,* pp. 41–43)

It is important to be aware of these symptoms, as your body is alerting you that something is not quite right.

FALSE TRUTHS

Arnold Fox, M.D., and Barry Fox, Ph.D., authors of *The Healthy Prostate,* claim that scientists don't actually know why the prostate begins to grow in later years. There are a number of theories that we will review in more detail in Chapter Two, along with the negative consequences of non-managed BPH. In a related note, Dr. Fox, an internist who also practices anti-aging medicine, insists that it is unfortunate that prostate disturbances have been categorized as a disease that only affects older men. According to Fox, prostate problems can strike at any age and new diagnostic procedures today suggest that many individuals suffering from prostate disturbances may have had the problem for years, never fully realizing it.

Andrew Weil, M.D., author of *Spontaneous Healing,* states that "the prostate gland is a vulnerable point of male anatomy, often harboring stubborn infections in youth and enlarging in age to the point of interfering with urination." (p. 260) Dr. Jeffrey L. Marrongelle, a chiropractor and certified nutritionist, maintains that once the key role in reproduction is mainly curtailed and the midlife marker of forty-five years is reached, the prostate seems to exist as a reservoir for toxins that accumulate in the body.

While the prostate's exact location may be a determining factor in some disorders, researchers believe that a combination of other factors—nutritional, environmental, hormonal, and stress-related—are all intertwined. In fact, many alternative healthcare providers maintain that these factors interfere with the body's inborn metabolic cycles. For example, Henry C. Bieler, M.D., one of the early medical professionals who pioneered the move toward natural non-invasive methods and their clinical application in the treatment of disease, maintained in his book, *Dr. Bieler's Natural Way to Sexual Health,* that, "the prostate gland is often used as an avenue of 'vicarious' elimination." (p. 87) Dr. Bieler points out that if you are extremely toxic and your liver and kidneys (the normal avenues of elimination) can't handle the overload of toxins, the prostate becomes a major dumping or holding site for these contaminates.

BREAKING THE CODE OF SILENCE

Although there is a continuing rise in the incidence of prostate dysfunction in many nations of the world, there still seems to be some unwritten code of silence about the subject throughout the male populations. In contrast, a large percentage of media attention centers on women's health issues—especially breast cancer. Michael Oppenheim, M.D., author of *The Man's Health Book,* points out that when you look at the covers of women's magazines you see women, and when you look at the cover of many men's magazines you see women again! Dr. Oppenheim maintains that men must learn to develop the same passion concerning their bodies and health as women do. This sentiment is echoed by Dr. Weil in his now-famous book, *8 Weeks to Optimum Health.* From his clinical experience, Weil believes that men disregard symptoms of illness and do not actively seek out help as quickly as females do. This trend is changing, however, due at least in part to the increasing number of men who have to deal with the long-term negative complications of prostate disorders. Men are beginning to actively and openly seek help and advice concerning the prostate's overall function. More importantly, males are looking for more preventive measures that will possibly slow down or forestall surgical or medical intervention.

Referring to high percentage of prostate disease in the U.S. population, Elliot Howard, M.D., of the Lenox Hill Hospital in

New York City, states, "You don't have to be on the wrong side of these statistics" amidst a society still intent on treatment versus prevention. The key is to learn as much as possible about how to keep the prostate gland healthy. After all, it is intimately involved with your sexual health as well as your general well-being.

Start by learning the warning signs associated with the different types of prostatic disorders. Moreover, if you are an African-American male, realize that you are much more susceptible to prostate disturbances. In fact, African-American males have the highest incidence of prostate cancer not only in the U.S. but in the world. In their own interest, black males must help to break this unwritten code of silence among men. Educating one another is a key variable in the fight to reducing the number of us who will suffer from complications associated with prostate malfunction.

SUMMARY

In 1987 about 96,000 cases of prostate cancer were diagnosed in the United States. In 1991, Dr. Howard Scher of the Memorial Sloan-Kettering Cancer Center in New York predicted that by the year 2000 there would be a ninety-percent increase in the annual occurrence of prostate disorders. Today, it is estimated that over twelve million men in the U.S. alone suffer from some sort of prostate disturbance. Although new cases of BPH are reported daily, the truth of the matter is that until this little gland starts acting up, many men still respond to the contention that it is the possible source of their problem with, *"Prostate who?"*

A couple of probing questions are put forth by Patrick C. Walsh, M.D., Chief of Urology at Johns Hopkins Hospital and Director of the Department of Urology at the Johns Hopkins University School of Medicine. Walsh asks:

1. Why do some men live for nearly a century without suffering from an enlarged prostate, while others, from middle age onward, need to be treated more than once?

2. Why do some men die with prostate cancer and others die of it, while other men never get the disease?

While certain physiological and biological changes, as well as the anatomical structure and location of the prostate gland, may pose some problems, living well and having a long-term maintenance plan in place may be the answer to the last question.

In the next chapter, "Understanding Prostate Disturbances," we will take an in-depth look at what can and will go wrong when one neglects good prostate health. Nature may not have provided long-term solutions for the prostate's care, but men can possibly offset or forestall impending problems by taking better care of themselves.

Please read on!

CHAPTER TWO

UNDERSTANDING PROSTATE DISTURBANCES

While the incidence of BPH is much more prevalent in the United States than in many foreign countries like Japan, this problem is one that affects millions of men around the world. One of the most discomforting symptoms of BPH is that normal sleep patterns can be constantly interrupted due to the necessity to void the bladder throughout the night. Matthew Hoffman and William LeGro, in their book *Disease Free*, describe the situation:

> Every night millions of. . . men with tired eyes and a brimming bladder leave the comfort of their bed to seek relief. No sooner do they settle back to sleep than their bladder, like an inexhaustible well, is full again. These uncomfortable fellows belong to what is perhaps the least exclusive club in the world: The Fraternal Order of Men with Enlarged Prostate Glands. (p. 430)

A more insidious problem associated with BPH is known as "silent prostatism." This disorder is characterized by urinary retention and a symptomatic obstruction of the release of urine. In other words, you may have the urge to urinate, but nothing flows out. As cited by Sandra Salmans, author of *Prostate Questions You Have . . . Answers You Need*, occasionally a man may not be aware he has an obstruction until it be-comes completely impossible for him to urinate." (pp. 52–53)

How can this happen and a man not be aware of it? This is the focus of Chapter Two. Here we will take a closer look at prostate dysfunction to gain a better understanding of the neg-ative ramifications of an enlarged prostate gland. In this chap-ter we will answer the following questions:

- ◆ What is BPH?
- ◆ What is prostatic obstruction and what are its signs?
- ◆ Does prostatic obstruction cause prostate cancer?
- ◆ How does it affect sexuality?
- ◆ What are the risk factors associated with BPH and prostate cancer?
- ◆ Why are African-American males more susceptible to pros-tate disturbances?
- ◆ When should a man seek professional help?
- ◆ What are the current treatment protocols for BPH and prostate cancer?
- ◆ Does heredity play a role in the onset of this disease?

As a holistic healthcare instructor and nutritional counselor, it still discourages me to find out how uniformed my male coun-terparts of all age groups are about their prostate gland and its health.

The old paradigm of the doctor telling the patient about the basic workings and care of the body is changing. People are taking more responsibility for their health. People like your wife and the women next door are learning how to better take care of themselves. You too, Mr. Male, need this same passion, drive, and enthusiasm for the care and basic operation of your body. Michael Colgan states "Clearly combating degenerative diseases is no longer the physician's battle, it is yours." (p. 20)

The goal of Chapter Two is to arm you with enough infor-mation to do just that—to prepare yourself for battle or a combative plan for prevention. Whichever action plan you choose, remember that you, the individual, can do more for your own health and well-being than any doctor, any hospital, drug or any exotic medical device.

BPH

As we learned in Chapter One, BPH stands for benign prostate hyperplasia. While BPH and the symptoms associated with cancer of the prostate gland are similar, having an enlarged prostate gland doesn't necessarily mean that you have prostate cancer. Benign means non-cancerous. Hyperplasia is a medical term used to describe an excessive growth of tissue. According to the National Cancer Institute, neither prostatitis (inflammation of the prostate) or prostate enlargement (BPH) is known to cause cancer.

If the growths are non-cancerous and are not life threatening, why all the concern? To answer that, take a minute to review the diagram of the prostate gland on page 5. As we discussed in Chapter One, the prostate gland wraps around the urethra, the narrow tube in the penis through which urine passes from the bladder, and this structure can sometimes pose problems from annoying to serious. Joseph E. Oesterling, M.D., Chief of Urology at the University of Michigan, and an authority on cancer of the prostate gland, reminds us that the prostate continues to grow throughout a man's life. When the prostate enlarges, it does so by expanding both outwardly and inwardly. (p. 6) This prostatic obstruction causes the prostate to squeeze the urethra too tightly, thus impeding the normal flow of urine from the body. Such a condition can possibly cause damage to the kidneys and lead to bladder stones, bleeding, and urinary tract infections.

STILL WATERS RUN DEEP

BPH is not like a common cold that will run its course. BPH and its silent onset can lead to full-blown blockage of the urethra.

If not treated, this can be fatal. Therefore, in this situation medical intervention is warranted immediately. Doctors will perform what is called a catherization. A tube known as a catheter is inserted through the penis into the bladder to let urine flow from the body.

It is vital that you know the warning signs of an enlarged prostate gland and possible obstruction of the urethra. To reiterate, those warning signs are:

- Frequent urge to urinate, especially at night
- Urge to urinate without any release of urine
- Decreased power in flow of urine stream
- Incontinence (loss of urinary control)
- Feeling that the bladder hasn't been completely emptied
- Painful or burning sensation during urination
- Straining to urinate
- Interruption of urine stream (starting and stopping of urine flow)
- Blood in the urine
- Uncontrolled urges toward sleep; weakness and irritability

While BPH does not usually affect sexual function itself, any painful ejaculation and/or blood in the ejaculate should send up a warning flag. According to Martin K. Gelband, M.D., a board-certified urologic surgeon and a Clinical Assistant Professor of Urology at the UCLA School of Medicine, painful ejaculation may be a sign of prostate inflammation and/or infection. Gelband goes on to say that while blood in the ejaculate may be an alarming sight, it rarely implies that a serious problem exists. Nevertheless, it should be checked out. Furthermore, reoccurring painful ejaculation plays a definite role in diminishing the desire to have sex. If, after appropriate testing, the condition comes up negative, hematospermia (blood in the ejaculate) that persists is usually treated with estrogen-like hormones. (pp. 205–206)

While both of these two occurrences should cause us to take note, blood in the urine will ring the alarm bell and have the urologist aggressively testing for the possibility that cancer of the prostate exists.

So, while BPH does not usually affect sexual function, this should not become your main determining factor in investigating the possibility that even the slight changes you are experiencing are just a temporary bump in the road. Rather, recognize that your body is talking to you loud and clear. Its silence has ended, and so should yours. Do not ignore it!

If you have had, or currently have, any of the above symptoms you should consult a urologist, a medical doctor who specializes in problems associated with the urinary tract.

SELF-TEST FOR BPH

To assist patients and their healthcare professional in determining just how severe BPH symptoms are, the American Urological Association has devised a questionnaire that will give you some indication of where you stand. While this is a subjective test—answers are based on your personal feelings—it can give you some indication as to whether medical intervention is warranted. If you are unsure or a little uncomfortable with your answers about how you physically feel, I strongly suggest that you talk with your personal physician.

Note: It is important that you understand the importance of checking with your medical professional, especially if your answers to the BPH self-test indicate you are in the severe range. If there is some underlying problem beyond benign prostate hyperplasia, the subjective test that follows cannot reveal and/or confirm it. Confirmation of cancer must be made by a biopsy, i.e., the diagnostic study of a piece of tissue from a living body.

WHAT'S CAUSING THE PROBLEM

There are numerous theories about the rising incidence of prostate disorders. These theories are called "known associated risk factors." Some of the risk factors linked to the cause of prostate disorders are:

SELF TEST FOR BPH

To help patients, and their physicians, assess the severity of BPH symptoms, the American Urological Association has developed a seven-question index.

Over the past month, how often have you:

1. _____ Had a sensation of not emptying your bladder completely after urinating?

2. _____ Had to urinate again less than two hours after urinating?

3. _____ Found you stopped and started again several times during urination?

4. _____ Found it difficult to postpone urination?

5. _____ Had a weak urinary stream?

6. _____ Had to push or strain to begin urination?

7. _____ Had to get up several times to urinate, from the time you went to bed at night until the time you got up in the morning (how many times)?

How To Score:

Questions 1–6: Give yourself a score of 1 for having problems less than one time in five, a score of 2 for having problems less than half the time, a score of 4 for having problems more than half the time, and a score of 5 for having problems almost all the time.

Question 7: Give yourself 1 for each time you got up in the night. (If you had to get up five times or more, use 5 for scoring.)

Mild Symptoms: Your score totals 1 to 7
Moderate Symptoms: Your score totals 8 to 19
Severe Symptoms: Your score totals 20 to 35

Source: National Cancer Institute Publication No. 98–4303, *Understanding Prostate Changes: A Health Guide for All Men*, Bethesda, Maryland, Sept. 1998, p.14.

- ◆ Stress
- ◆ Aging
- ◆ Nationality
- ◆ Obesity
- ◆ High fat diets
- ◆ Consumption of red meats
- ◆ Heredity
- ◆ Metabolic disturbances
- ◆ Exposure to pesticides
- ◆ Your occupation
- ◆ Where you live
- ◆ Hormonal changes
- ◆ Sexual inactivity
- ◆ What country you live in

This list represents only a small portion of the associated risk factors in the development of prostate disorders. Age is probably the most predominant factor. Ann Louise Gittleman, M.S., author of *Super Nutrition for Men and the Women Who Love Them,* writes: "By age fifty 30% of all males begin to experience symptoms of BPH. By sixty, half will be affected. Beyond age seventy, almost 80% will develop this disorder. And by age eighty almost every man in the U.S. will have BPH." (p. 60)

Where you live is one of the associated risk factors that researchers are exploring more aggressively today. In the U.S., for instance, prostate disturbances occur at much higher rates in certain parts of the country as demonstrated in Figure 2.1.

MY COUNTRY 'TIS OF THEE

Prostate dysfunction is not limited to any one country. However, where you live in the world seems to have some bearing on the statistical incidence of men who suffer from this malady. (See Figure 2.2)

The data indicates a possible link between lifestyle (within a particular country) and the rising incidence and severity of prostate disorders. From Figure 2.2 we can see that the lowest mortality rates from prostate cancer are among Asian men. The highest incidence is in Switzerland (22.0) and the Nordic countries (17.7–21.2).

While the United States falls in the middle range (15.7), look at Thailand. Their rate, 0.2 means that only 0.2 males out of every 100,000 contract prostate cancer, or one man in 500,000.

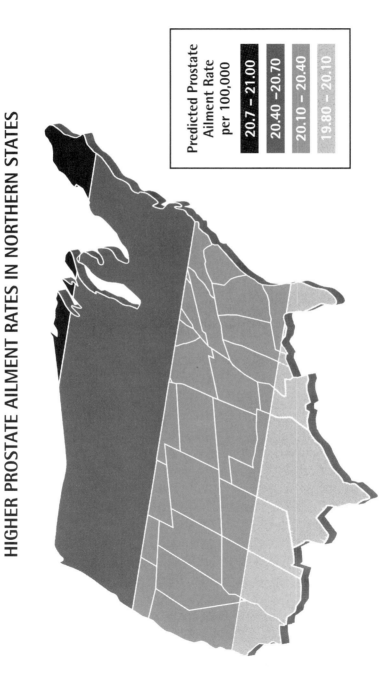

HIGHER PROSTATE AILMENT RATES IN NORTHERN STATES

Predicted Prostate
Ailment Rate
per 100,000

20.7 – 21.00
20.40 – 20.70
20.10 – 20.40
19.80 – 20.10

Figure 2.1 Source: *Prostate Health without Drugs or Surgery*, Gero-Vita Laboratories, Toronto, Ontario, Canada, p.4. Used with permission.

PROSTATE CANCER DEATH RATES
Among 50 Countries

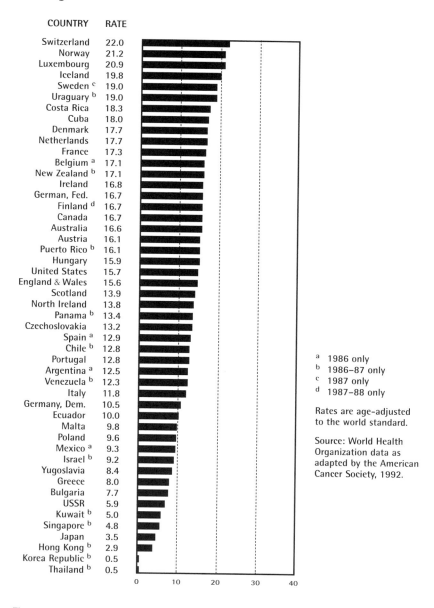

COUNTRY	RATE
Switzerland	22.0
Norway	21.2
Luxembourg	20.9
Iceland	19.8
Sweden [c]	19.0
Uraguary [b]	19.0
Costa Rica	18.3
Cuba	18.0
Denmark	17.7
Netherlands	17.7
France	17.3
Belgium [a]	17.1
New Zealand [b]	17.1
Ireland	16.8
German, Fed.	16.7
Finland [d]	16.7
Canada	16.7
Australia	16.6
Austria	16.1
Puerto Rico [b]	16.1
Hungary	15.9
United States	15.7
England & Wales	15.6
Scotland	13.9
North Ireland	13.8
Panama [b]	13.4
Czechoslovakia	13.2
Spain [a]	12.9
Chile [b]	12.8
Portugal	12.8
Argentina [a]	12.5
Venezuela [b]	12.3
Italy	11.8
Germany, Dem.	10.5
Ecuador	10.0
Malta	9.8
Poland	9.6
Mexico [a]	9.3
Israel [b]	9.2
Yugoslavia	8.4
Greece	8.0
Bulgaria	7.7
USSR	5.9
Kuwait [b]	5.0
Singapore [b]	4.8
Japan	3.5
Hong Kong [b]	2.9
Korea Republic [b]	0.5
Thailand [b]	0.5

[a] 1986 only
[b] 1986–87 only
[c] 1987 only
[d] 1987–88 only

Rates are age-adjusted
to the world standard.

Source: World Health
Organization data as
adapted by the American
Cancer Society, 1992.

Figure 2.2 Source: *Cancer Rates and Risks,* National Institutes of Health, National Cancer Institutes, Bethesda Maryland, 4th ed., 1996, p.45. Used with permission. [*Death Rates per 100,000 population, male.*]

Based on data compiled by the World Health Organization and cited by the National Cancer Institute in the United States, Thailand also has the lowest incidence of lung, breast, stomach, and cervical cancer. In fact, current data shows that Thailand and several other less developed nations have significantly lower rates of cancer, outpacing the United States by leaps and bounds. (See Figures 2.3 and 2.4)

Why such a difference between Thailand, for instance, and the U.S.? In subsequent chapters we will take a closer look at this phenomenon, examining the products, nutritional preferences, and lifestyles within these countries to see how they correlate with the statistics represented here.

THE AFRICAN-AMERICAN CONNECTION

African-American males have higher rates of prostate cancer than any other group of U.S males, and any other group of males in the world. In 1991, data complied by the National Cancer Institute revealed that 25 out of every 100,000 African-American men died of prostate cancer. The chances of black males developing this disease is thrity-two percent higher than that of American whites. In a related matter, at a recent conference held in Washington D.C. (January, 1998), Dr. Charles J. McDonald, then president-elect of the American Cancer Society, made note that for black men in America the risk of developing prostate cancer was rising. In 1998, according to Dr. McDonald, for every 100,000 black men, an estimated 234 would be diagnosed with cancer of the prostate gland compared to 135 out of every 100,000 white American males. He went on to say that black men are two to three times more likely to die of the disease. (pp. 24–25)

THE SEER PROGRAM

As a result of the rising incidence of cancer in the United States and the need to establish and understand why cancers seem to develop more often in some groups, the National Cancer Act of 1971 mandated the collection, analysis, and dissemination of information that could help prevent, properly diagnose, and treat different forms of cancer.

An outgrowth of this mandate was the formation of the Surveillance, Epidemiology and End Results (SEER) Program. As a continuing project of the National Cancer Institute, the SEER Program is responsible for monitoring the impact of cancer in the general population of the United States. The following charts (Figures 2.5–2.8) give a detailed analysis of the variation of racial and ethnic incidences of prostate cancer.

The first graph, SEER Incidence Rates Among Men, shows that the occurrences of prostate cancer among black men (180.6 per 100,000) is more than seven times that of Korean men (24.2). The ratio for white males is also quite high. (See Figure 2.5 and 2.6)

Figure 2.7 shows prostate incidence rates of cancer by age, while Figure 2.8 shows U.S. mortality rates of men by age at death.

THE TESTOSTERONE STORY

Scientists have discovered a strong link in the development of prostate disturbances with overproduction of the hormone testosterone. While women have low levels of this hormone, the testicles and adrenal glands in men produce the testosterone that promotes male sex drive, muscularity and physical prowess. Aging causes a natural decline in the production of this hormone. However, researchers have discovered that dihydrotestosterone—an extremely potent hormone the body produces from testosterone—causes cells in the prostate to multiply out of control, thus causing the prostate gland to enlarge. One of the medical treatments for prostate enlargement, which we will cover in more detail in Chapter Three, is the use of medications to slowdown the production of testosterone.

The higher incidence of prostate disorders, including cancer, in African-American males is due to the fact that they produce up to fifteen percent more testosterone that white males. Health professionals believe that this is a major reason why African-American males develop prostate disorders, especially

CANCER DEATH RATES—MALES

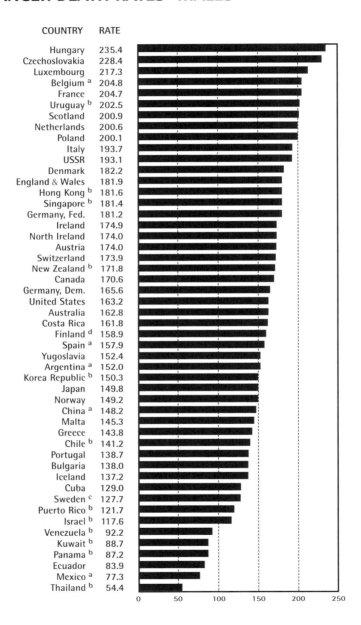

COUNTRY	RATE
Hungary	235.4
Czechoslovakia	228.4
Luxembourg	217.3
Belgium [a]	204.8
France	204.7
Uruguay [b]	202.5
Scotland	200.9
Netherlands	200.6
Poland	200.1
Italy	193.7
USSR	193.1
Denmark	182.2
England & Wales	181.9
Hong Kong [b]	181.6
Singapore [b]	181.4
Germany, Fed.	181.2
Ireland	174.9
North Ireland	174.0
Austria	174.0
Switzerland	173.9
New Zealand [b]	171.8
Canada	170.6
Germany, Dem.	165.6
United States	163.2
Australia	162.8
Costa Rica	161.8
Finland [d]	158.9
Spain [a]	157.9
Yugoslavia	152.4
Argentina [a]	152.0
Korea Republic [b]	150.3
Japan	149.8
Norway	149.2
China [a]	148.2
Malta	145.3
Greece	143.8
Chile [b]	141.2
Portugal	138.7
Bulgaria	138.0
Iceland	137.2
Cuba	129.0
Sweden [c]	127.7
Puerto Rico [b]	121.7
Israel [b]	117.6
Venezuela [b]	92.2
Kuwait [b]	88.7
Panama [b]	87.2
Ecuador	83.9
Mexico [a]	77.3
Thailand [b]	54.4

Figure 2.3 Source: *Cancer Rates and Risk.* National Institute of Health, National Cancer Institute, Bethesda Maryland, 4th ed, 1996, p.39. Used with Permission. [*Death Rates per 100,000 population male.*]

CANCER DEATH RATES–FEMALES

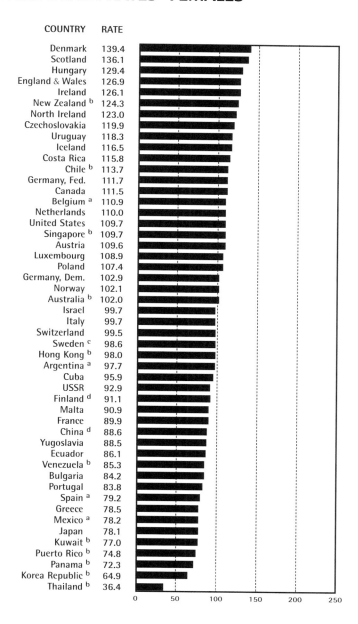

COUNTRY	RATE
Denmark	139.4
Scotland	136.1
Hungary	129.4
England & Wales	126.9
Ireland	126.1
New Zealand [b]	124.3
North Ireland	123.0
Czechoslovakia	119.9
Uruguay	118.3
Iceland	116.5
Costa Rica	115.8
Chile [b]	113.7
Germany, Fed.	111.7
Canada	111.5
Belgium [a]	110.9
Netherlands	110.0
United States	109.7
Singapore [b]	109.7
Austria	109.6
Luxembourg	108.9
Poland	107.4
Germany, Dem.	102.9
Norway	102.1
Australia [b]	102.0
Israel	99.7
Italy	99.7
Switzerland	99.5
Sweden [c]	98.6
Hong Kong [b]	98.0
Argentina [a]	97.7
Cuba	95.9
USSR	92.9
Finland [d]	91.1
Malta	90.9
France	89.9
China [d]	88.6
Yugoslavia	88.5
Ecuador	86.1
Venezuela [b]	85.3
Bulgaria	84.2
Portugal	83.8
Spain [a]	79.2
Greece	78.5
Mexico [a]	78.2
Japan	78.1
Kuwait [b]	77.0
Puerto Rico [b]	74.8
Panama [b]	72.3
Korea Republic [b]	64.9
Thailand [b]	36.4

Figure 2.4 Source: *Cancer Rates and Risk.* National Institute of Health, National Cancer Institute, Bethesda Maryland, 4th ed, 1996, p.39. Used with Permission. [*Death Rates per 100,000 population female.*]

SEER INCIDENCE RATES: Among Men, 1988–1992

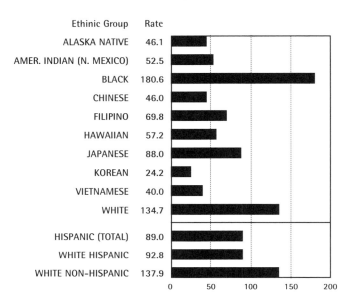

Ethinic Group	Rate	
ALASKA NATIVE	46.1	
AMER. INDIAN (N. MEXICO)	52.5	
BLACK	180.6	
CHINESE	46.0	
FILIPINO	69.8	
HAWAIIAN	57.2	
JAPANESE	88.0	
KOREAN	24.2	
VIETNAMESE	40.0	
WHITE	134.7	
HISPANIC (TOTAL)	89.0	
WHITE HISPANIC	92.8	
WHITE NON-HISPANIC	137.9	

Figure 2.5 Source: "Racial/Ethnic Patterns of Cancer in United States," SEER Monograph, National Cancer Institute, Bethesda Maryland, May 1998, p.109. *[Rates are "average annual" per 100,00 population, age-adjusted to 1970 U.S. standard; N/A = information not available: * = rate not calculated when fewer than 25 cases.]*

cancer, much earlier in life. According to David G. Bostwick, M.D., an expert in disorders of the prostate gland, the death rate from prostate cancer of black males in the U.S. far exceeds that of black males in East Africa. This suggests again that the lifestyles of American men, regardless of race, plays a major role in the onset and the long-term development of prostate disturbances.

If you are a black male, you must help break this unwritten code of silence about prostate disorders. To aid in this battle, the Fox Chase Cancer Center in Philadelphia has established a nationwide preventive program for African-American males between the ages of thirty-five and sixty-nine ("Men's Health

U.S. MORTALITY RATES: Among Men, 1988–1992

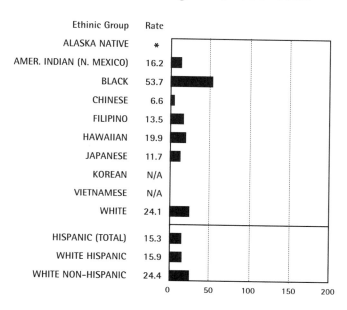

Figure 2.6 Source: "Racial/Ethnic Patterns of Cancer in United States," SEER Monograph, National Cancer Institute, Bethesda Maryland, May 1998, p.109. [*Rates are "average annual" per 100,00 population, age-adjusted to 1970 U.S. standard; N/A = information not available: * = rate not calculated when fewer than 25 cases.*]

Alert," *Community Service Bulletin*) For more information call 215-728-2406 or 888-Fox Chase. You can also visit their website at *http://www.feec.edu.web*

Information concerning other websites and facilities in the U.S. and around the world can be found in Chapter Nine, "Getting The Help You Need."

THE SILENT KILLER

Much like diabetes, high blood pressure, and heart disease, the inception, progression and imminent development of prostate cancer can go undetected for years. In fact, prostate cancer

SEER INCIDENCE RATES
Among Men by Age at Diagnosis, 1988–1992

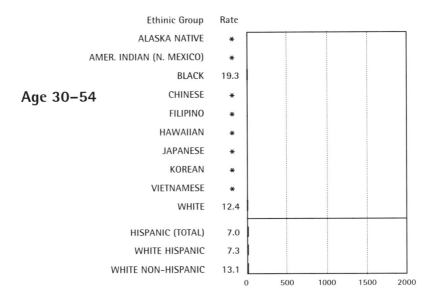

Ethinic Group	Rate
ALASKA NATIVE	*
AMER. INDIAN (N. MEXICO)	*
BLACK	19.3
CHINESE	*
FILIPINO	*
HAWAIIAN	*
JAPANESE	*
KOREAN	*
VIETNAMESE	*
WHITE	12.4
HISPANIC (TOTAL)	7.0
WHITE HISPANIC	7.3
WHITE NON-HISPANIC	13.1

Age 30–54

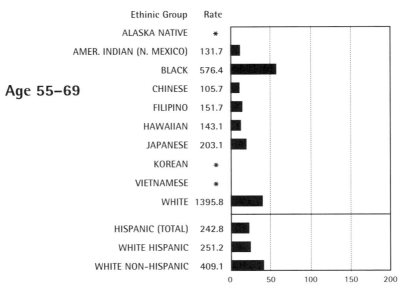

Ethinic Group	Rate
ALASKA NATIVE	*
AMER. INDIAN (N. MEXICO)	131.7
BLACK	576.4
CHINESE	105.7
FILIPINO	151.7
HAWAIIAN	143.1
JAPANESE	203.1
KOREAN	*
VIETNAMESE	*
WHITE	1395.8
HISPANIC (TOTAL)	242.8
WHITE HISPANIC	251.2
WHITE NON-HISPANIC	409.1

Age 55–69

continued

SEER INCIDENCE RATES   *continued*
Among Men by Age at Diagnosis, 1988–1992

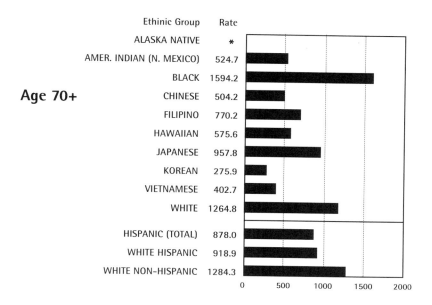

Figure 2.7 Source: "Racial/Ethnic Patterns of Cancer in United States," SEER Monograph, National Cancer Institute, Bethesda Maryland, May 1998, p.110. *[Rates are per 100,000 population, age adjusted to 1970 U.S. standard; *= rate not calculated when fewer than 25 cases.]*

grows very slowly—so slowly, that many men in their seventies and eighties die with prostate cancer. When it spreads beyond the prostate itself, this cancer can be very aggressive.

Johns Hopkins urologist Patrick C. Walsh, M.D., states:

> For too many men, death from prostate cancer is a sad end to months of excruciating pain, increasingly thin and brittle, cancer-riddled bones, awful constipation from pain-killing drugs, and miserable symptoms of urinary obstruction. (p. 23)

Early detection is vital. However, because signs and symptoms of prostate cancer do not always manifest themselves, in many cases by the time a man shows outward signs of prostate cancer, curing it becomes very difficult, if not impossible. (p. 37)

U.S. MORTALITY RATES
Among Men by Age at Death, 1988–1992

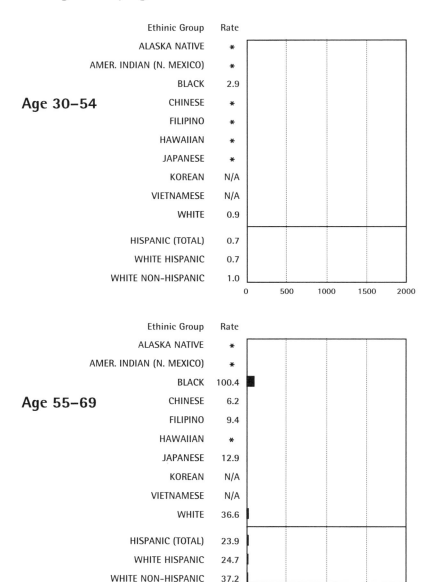

Age 30–54

Ethinic Group	Rate
ALASKA NATIVE	*
AMER. INDIAN (N. MEXICO)	*
BLACK	2.9
CHINESE	*
FILIPINO	*
HAWAIIAN	*
JAPANESE	*
KOREAN	N/A
VIETNAMESE	N/A
WHITE	0.9
HISPANIC (TOTAL)	0.7
WHITE HISPANIC	0.7
WHITE NON-HISPANIC	1.0

0   500   1000   1500   2000

Age 55–69

Ethinic Group	Rate
ALASKA NATIVE	*
AMER. INDIAN (N. MEXICO)	*
BLACK	100.4
CHINESE	6.2
FILIPINO	9.4
HAWAIIAN	*
JAPANESE	12.9
KOREAN	N/A
VIETNAMESE	N/A
WHITE	36.6
HISPANIC (TOTAL)	23.9
WHITE HISPANIC	24.7
WHITE NON-HISPANIC	37.2

0   50   100   150   200

continued

U.S. MORTALITY RATES   *continued*
Among Men by Age at Death, 1988–1992

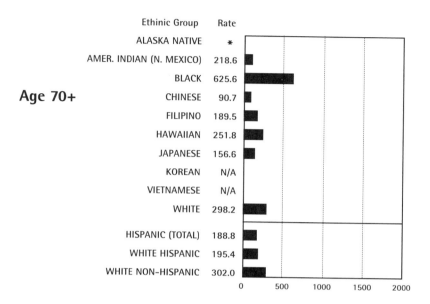

Ethinic Group	Rate
ALASKA NATIVE	*
AMER. INDIAN (N. MEXICO)	218.6
BLACK	625.6
CHINESE	90.7
FILIPINO	189.5
HAWAIIAN	251.8
JAPANESE	156.6
KOREAN	N/A
VIETNAMESE	N/A
WHITE	298.2
HISPANIC (TOTAL)	188.8
WHITE HISPANIC	195.4
WHITE NON–HISPANIC	302.0

Age 70+

Figure 2.8 Source: "Racial/Ethnic Patterns of Cancer in United States," SEER Monograph, National Cancer Institute, Bethesda Maryland, May 1998, p.111. [*Rates are per 100,000 population, age adjusted to 1970 U.S. standard; *=rate not calculated when fewer than 25 cases.*]

HEREDITY

To fully understand prostate disturbances, it is important to also realize that your genes could have a hand it all of this. According to researchers at Fox Chase Cancer Center, many males are totally unaware of their inherited risk of developing prostate cancer. If other men in your family have had prostate disease, your chances of developing this malady increase. This is due to your inherited DNA structure. (DNA is the basic biologically-active chemical in humans and nearly all living organisms that determines their physical development, growth and repair.) Since genetic alterations in cells tend to occur with advancing age, most disorders, like prostate cancer, tend to develop later in life.

In a related matter, researchers at the Brady Urological Institute at Johns Hopkins emphasized to doctors there the importance of taking into consideration family members on both sides of a patient's family. The health history of fathers, brothers, uncles, and grandfathers on both sides of a family is invaluable information since chances of developing prostate cancer increase eight times the normal average if any two first-line relatives has had the disease.

Data of this nature has led some researchers, including Stuart Berger, M.D., winner of the George W. Thorn Award for extraordinary professional accomplishment, to conclude that, "Life is a terminal disease. The human body is programmed to self-destruct and the code to do so is written in our genes." (p. 40) Dr. Berger is known as a "genetic fatalist."

Berger's train of thought, is being challenged by other health professionals, such as Deepak Chopra, Andrew Weil, and Robert Atkins—all medical doctors specializing in alternative medicine—who stress that you are not simply a victim of your genes. Nutritional researchers such as Victoria Dolby Toews, M.P.H., maintain that you can take action to protect the 100 trillion or so cells in your body, and such action is paramount in the quest for vibrant health. "Strengthening and maintaining the structural integrity of cells (and protecting their precious cargo: DNA) increases our resistance to disease and helps protect us against gene-altering diseases, such as cancer." (p. 36)

KNOWLEDGE IS POWER

You have the ability to eliminate or slow down the destructive forces of prostate disease. For example, researchers now know that diets high in animal fat and the consumption of red meat can dramatically increase testosterone levels in the body—a major reason why prostate cancer seems to flourish in countries where diets are high in the consumption of red meat and animal fats. This you control!

To get a clearer picture of some of the risk factors discussed here, as well as others, please refer to Appendix A, "Know Your Prostate Cancer Risk Factors," at the back of this book. Take a moment to complete a short test there to measure your prostate cancer risk. Between this and the self-test for BPH contained in Chapter One, you should have a better overall picture of where you stand.

Note: Consult with your healthcare professional about your concerns and questions.

THE SIGNS OF PROSTATE CANCER

The signs and symptoms of BPH are the same for established signs of prostate cancer. A few additional symptoms of prostate cancer, including pain in the lower back or pelvic area, loss of appetite and weight loss, should be cause for investigation. These signs and symptoms may not mean that you have cancer, but it is important to check with your healthcare professional to rule out its possibility.

I strongly recommend that you follow the established guidelines concerning examinations and early detection of prostate cancer. They are:

1. Starting at age forty, men should have yearly digital rectal exams (DRE).

2. At age fifty (or ages thirty-five to forty if there is a history of prostate cancer in your family) annual blood tests for prostate-specific antigen (PSA) should be begun.

We will cover more about diagnosis and treatment options in Chapter Three. For now, keep in mind that the more you understand about prostate disorders, the easier it will be to develop a plan of action toward prevention.

Break this code of silence, as every three minutes a new case of prostate cancer is diagnosed in the United States, and every thirteen minutes a man dies of this disease. When it comes to cancer of the prostate, an ounce of prevention is definitely worth more than a pound of cure.

IT'S NOT ELEMENTARY, WATSON

Now that you have a clearer understanding of how and why prostate disturbances occur, the question then becomes, what is the best way to treat them?

As we continue to dig a little deeper you will find that much controversy exists regarding the best way to treat prostate dysfunction in its many forms and degrees of severity. In fact, if you were to go to several different urologists for the same problem, you might be surprised to find that each doctor could suggest a different approach.

In the next chapter, "The Treatment Options," we will take a look at the many protocols available, both conventional and alternative. Although researchers are unsure whether the primary factor in prostate disorders is genetics, lifestyle, or environmental concerns, deciding how to treat the negative symptoms associated with this disorder raises complex issues. Whatever the treatment decision, it is a foregone conclusion that it's anything but elementary.

CHAPTER THREE

DIAGNOSING PROSTATE DISTURBANCES

Back in the 1950s, there were few tools to assist in diagnosing prostate problems. We've come a long way since then, and now we have a wide variety of diagnostic tests and procedures that can help us diagnose prostate problems.

—*Arnold Fox, M.D.,* and *Barry Fox, Ph.D.*

Mainstream medical professionals today employ a number of treatments for prostate disorders ranging from radical prostatectomy, cryosurgery, and external beam radiation, to radioactive seed implants. Alternative healthcare practitioners—like Dr. Robert Atkins, Michael Murray, N.D., of Bastyr University in Seattle; Harry C. Preuss, M.D., at Georgetown University Medical Center; and Kurt W. Donsbach, Ph.D., N.D., of the Hospital Santa Monica (Rosarito, Mexico)—contend that prostate disturbances will in many cases respond to hyperthermia (heat applied to an enlarged prostate), as well as to nutritional and other herbal and natural remedies. In fact, Dr. Atkins states that "Prostate enlargement responds so well to nutritional and herbal medicine that mainstream solutions are in fact completely unnecessary." (p. 349)

Despite the sophistication of treatment protocols available, many conventional doctors are still unsure if any surgical procedures actually extend or improve the quality of life of most of their patients, more than would non-treatment and/or watch-ful waiting. Dr. Jay Goldstein, who has had residences in both psychiatry and family medicine at the University of California and who is known as the "Doctor of Last Resort," states that "Unless your problem has clear medical-cookbook symptoms and responds to medical-cookbook treatment, many (perhaps most) physicians don't really want to deal with it—or with you." He goes on to say that "If it's not in the cookbook, most doctors seem to say it doesn't exist." Goldstein points out that most physicians rarely question that "the cookbook" itself could be inadequate. (p. 2)

THE DIAGNOSTIC PROCESS

A number of tests are commonly employed today to deter-mine the overall health of the prostate gland. They include:

1. The Digital Rectal Exam (DRE)
2. Prostate–specific antigen (PSA)
3. Transrectal ultrasound (TRUS)
4. The biopsy
5. The Gleason Scale

1. The Digital Rectal Exam (DRE)

This is the standard physical method used to assess the condi-tion of the prostate gland. In this exam, your physician will ask you to stand and bend forward, at which time the doctor will insert a lubricated gloved finger into the rectum. The doctor is feeling for lumps, enlargement, or hard areas of the prostate that could possibly mean the presence of cancer, since the prostate gland is usually soft and rubbery.

Because of the proximity of the prostate gland to the rectum, the DRE allows your physician to easily determine the pros-tate's firmness and texture. This test only takes a minute and should become routine during yearly exams, especially if you are forty or older.

Although the DRE is a standard evaluation tool, it does have some drawbacks. According to Don Kaltenbach, president and founder of the Prostate Cancer Resource Network and winner of the American Cancer Society's Media Award for his book *Prostate Cancer: A Survivor's Guide,* the results of the digital rectal exam are inconclusive and sometimes not very accurate because the exam only allows the posterior portion of the prostate gland to be felt. (p. 2)

2. The Prostate–Specific Antigen Test (PSA)

Because of the shortcomings of the digital rectal exam, a test commonly known as the PSA, which stands for prostate-specific antigen, is measured via a blood test. PSA is a protein manufactured only by the cells of the prostate gland.

When the prostate gland begins to enlarge, PSA levels in the blood are elevated. The presence of cancer also can cause PSA levels to rise. Prostatitis (inflammation of the prostate gland) can also cause PSA levels to be elevated temporarily.

All in all, when the digital rectal exam and the prostate-specific antigen blood test are used together as an evaluation tool, they are excellent indicators of the health of the prostate gland.

Note: A PSA blood test that shows a blood range of 0 to 4.0 ng/ml (nonograms per milliliter of blood) is considered normal. Scores between 4 and 10 are considered slightly elevated. Scores in this range do not necessarily indicate cancer, according to Kent Wallner, M.D., of the Memorial Sloan-Kettering Center, New York. However, in some cases doctors will suggest that a biopsy be done to rule out that possibility.

Scores of 10 to 20, or 20 and above, are considered suspicious and warrant further testing.

3. Transrectal Ultrasound

In this procedure a tiny probe is inserted into the rectum. The probe emits and picks up high-frequency sound waves, much like the ultrasound that pregnant women receive when they wish to view their baby. The sound waves produced by healthy tissue and cancerous prostate tissue are distinctly different.

This test is very useful when following up on questionable DRE and PSA tests.

4. The Biopsy

When in doubt, to be one hundred percent sure of a diagnosis your doctor will order a biopsy. The biopsy involves the extraction of tissue samples from the prostate gland. This is the only method that can absolutely verify the presence or non-presence of cancer.

5. The Gleason Score

Once a biopsy is done, a pathologist will study the results found. Pathologists use a method called the Gleason Score to determine the health of the prostate gland. The scale runs from 2 to 10. Scores of 2, 3, 4 are considered good, meaning that although cancer may be present, it remains localized within the prostate gland itself.

Scores of 8, 9, 10 are considered bad, meaning that there is a strong possibility that the cancer has spread to other parts of the body.

A score right in the middle creates a dilemma, according to Dr. Walsh at Johns Hopkins. Because prostate cancers are slow growing and may never become a serious threat to health, a mid-range score poses decision problems in reference to treatment. In such a situation, Dr. Martin Gelbard at the UCLA School of Medicine maintains that the primary criterion for choosing observation or "watchful waiting" rather than aggressive treatment (radiation or surgery) would be a slow growth rate of localized cancer, and the life expectancy of the patient. (p. 149)

While the scope of this book cannot cover all aspects of the diagnosis of prostate problems, the five methods listed above represent the common protocols in evaluating prostate health. When treatment beyond that of watchful waiting is warranted, there are many other options that can be explored. Many of the conventional treatments used are based on the staging sequence of prostate cancer. Staging represents the severity of a particular situation. For example, Stage A cancers are usually confined to the prostate, and can't be detected by a DRE. They usually produce no signs or symptoms at all. Stage B cancer is usually found within the prostate capsule and has not mestastized. It can be detected by a DRE. [**Note:** According to Dr. Kent Wallner, death from stage A or B prostate cancer within ten years of diagnosis is highly unlikely. There is, however, the risk that the cancer may spread. (p. 37)] Stage C cancer has extended beyond the prostate gland with visible outward signs. Stage D may have spread to the seminal vesicle and lymph nodes, and perhaps to the liver, bones or other tissues. [**Note:** Other sophisticated tests such as bone scans, CAT scans, and MRI's (magnetic resonance imaging) are also employed to determine the severity of the diagnosis.]

Once the magnitude of an individual prostate problem has been defined and staged, treatment options are then decided upon. At this point, keep in mind the advice of Dr. Arnold Fox,

> Physicians are great for helping you discover what may be going wrong inside your body, as well as for suggesting treatments. But only you should make the choice to pursue medical or surgical treatment. Remember, all medicines and surgeries harbor some danger, and should be approached with healthy caution. Even a small chance of side effects may be too great if you're the one who has to live with them. (p. ix)

As Dr. Fox indicates, you must take into consideration your age, the stage of your problem, your PSA and Gleason score, as well as the results of your digital rectal exam. In treating BPH, watchful waiting, especially in those of you with mild symptoms, may be suggested. In some cases, however, medication or surgery may be recommended. It is very important, however, that you participate actively in your health program every step of the way. This is where many of the alternative treatments used today can be of great benefit, due in part to their preventive as well as restorative capabilities. Many aternative protocols are excellent adjuncts to standard conventional treatments and, depending on the severity of your prostate dysfunction, can be viable options. Please check with your healthcare professional before choosing or eliminating any current treatment plan.

Furthermore, researchers at the National Cancer Institute maintain that for most men there is no "right answer." They strongly recommend that you make your own decisions, taking into account the advice of your doctor and the best, most up-to-date information that you can gather.

To assist you in this process please refer to Appendix B at the end of this book. The section entitled "How to Decipher the Idiosyncrasies of Scientific Reporting" will show you how to interpret the scientific jargon in the reports and studies that you may come across in your investigation.

BE AN INFORMED CONSUMER

If you know how your illness can affect your body, and if you stay informed about the progress of your treatment, you have a better chance to take part in your care. Learn as much as you can about what is happening to you. If you have questions, ask your doctor and other members of your treatment team. Your pharmacist is a good person to talk to if you have questions about your medicines. If you don't understand the answer to a question, ask it again.

Some patients hesitate to ask their doctors about their treatment options. They may think that doctors do not like to have their recommendations questioned. Most doctors, however, believe that the best patient is an informed patient. They understand that coping with treatment is easier when patients understand as much as possible, and they encourage patients to discuss their concerns.

When you see your doctor to talk about possible treatments or to get help for problems that come up during treatment, take your list of questions and ask a friend or relative to go with you. You'll get the most useful advice if you and your companion speak openly with the doctor about your needs, expectations, wishes and concerns.

Taking an active part in your care can help you have a sense of control, well-being, and a positive mental outlook toward the future.

In the next chapter, "Conventional Treatments," we will consider many of the treatment protocols suggested by allopathic practitioners.

PART TWO

The Treatment Options

Many physicians feel that surgery is the only solution to prostate problems. However, benign prostatic hyperplasia will often respond to nutritional and herbal support. This is particularly important as the surgical procedure often results in complications.

—*Michael Murray, N.D.,*
and *Joseph Pizzorno, N.D.*

THE TREATMENT OPTIONS

One hundred years ago the main treatment for men who suffered from obstruction of urine flow due to BPH was castration. Since the cause of BPH was associated with the overproduction of the male hormone testosterone, castration was a way to stop the hormone secretion. Researchers had learned that the epithelial cells that line the ducts within the prostate actually caused the prostate to enlarge. The culprit causing this enlargement was dihydrotestosterone (DHT). Dihydrotestosterone is converted from testosterone by an enzyme known as 5-alpha reductase by the cells found within the prostate gland itself.

Today, medical professionals employ the use of different drugs to counter the production of testosterone. The drug Finasteride, commonly known as Proscar™, actually inhibits the action of the enzyme 5-alpha reductase. Although Proscar™ is widely prescribed today, it does have some side effects, as do most drugs. Decreased libido, ejaculatory problems, and impotency are the most common. Also, women who are pregnant are warned against handling the tablets. Even when they are not ingested, contact with them can cause birth abnormalities in an unborn fetus.

On the other side of the coin, alternative healthcare professionals have found that natural sterols (compounds naturally occurring in plants) found in the herb *Serenoa repens,* commonly known as saw palmetto, lessen the severity of problems associated with BPH. The action of this non-pharmacological extract is the same as that of Proscar™. The sterols in saw palmetto also block the conversion of testosterone to dihydrotestosterone. In head to head trials, saw palmetto has outpaced Proscar™ in its ability to slow down the progression of an enlarged prostate gland, and without the side effects. In Chapter Six we will cover in more detail the attributes of natural supplements. The goal of Part Two of this book is to present as much up-to-date information as possible concerning conventional as well as alternative treatment options.

CHAPTER FOUR

CONVENTIONAL TREATMENTS

Treatment of prostate cancer is one of the most controversial areas in medicine.

—Kent Wallner, M.D.

Along with the prominent doctors already quoted, Dr. Kent Wallner, who has authored over sixty scientific articles on prostate cancer and its treatment, suggests that "watchful waiting" should be explored before surgical intervention is undertaken. Dr. Wallner also notes that when treatment for a prostate disorder becomes necessary, you will probably get many different opinions as to which treatment mode would be best.

This same sentiment is expressed by Sandra Salmans, author of *Prostate Questions You Have... Answers You Need.* A former staff writer for the *New York Times* and *Newsweek,* Salmans states that "If you consult with more than one doctor you may get more than one different opinion." She goes on to say that considerable disagreement exists within medical circles about which treatments are most effective." (p. 159)

The bottom line here is that *you the individual* should be familiar with what treatment plans or protocols are available. Also, it is critical that you thoroughly understand the pros and cons of each therapy. I cannot stress this fact enough. Doctors, like everyone else, have biases which have nothing to do with you as an individual patient, but apply to the doctor's area of expertise. Simply speaking, doctors tend to recommend what they know how to do. Surgeons tend to suggest surgery, while a radiation oncologist will usually propose the use of radiation.

CONVENTIONAL TREATMENTS

This section gives you an overview of some of the most widely used conventional medical treatments for various stages of prostate disturbance.

Chemotherapy

Chemotherapy involves the use of toxic drugs to kill cancer cells. Chemotherapy, while it attacks cancerous cells, is poisonous to all types of cells, meaning that in the process of treatment many normal cells are destroyed. Only about twenty percent of prostate cancer tumors will shrink via chemotherapy and, according to Dr. Wallner, the shrinkage lasts only about two months. In essence, this therapy may only cause a temporary remission of this disease. (pp. 139–140)

Cryosurgery (Cryo)

Cryosurgery, or "cryo" as it is commonly called, is performed by inserting three to six coreless needles into the prostate gland. With the assistance of an ultrasound machine, the surgeon guides the placement of these needles. Once in place they freeze the prostate. Freezing causes prostate gland tissue to die. This dead tissue is harmlessly absorbed by the body.

One of the problems with cryosurgery is the risk of urinary incontinence in two to ten percent of men in the first year after treatment. (Wallner, p. 118) Although cryosurgery is not new, it is new in the treatment of prostate disorders.

External Beam Radiation Therapy

The major focus of this treatment is to halt the progression of cancer cell growth. A "Star Wars"-type machine called a linear accelerator radiates beams of radiation to precise sites on the external surface. The beam gives off high doses of radiation which penetrate through the skin to attack cancer cells.

This procedure has a good cure rate for prostate cancer in its early stages; however, it carries the risk of damaging healthy tissue and may cause side effects such as diarrhea, upset stomach, impotence and urinary incontinence. This treatment is often recommended for older men because, as a non-surgical intervention, it eliminates the complications, including the risk of death, that may accompany surgery. However, the major concern with radiation therapy is that there is still considerable doubt following treatment that the cancer has been totally eradicated.

Orchiectomy (Castration)

As we learned, castration is a surgical procedure involving the removal of the testicles. In medical terms the procedure is known as an orchiectomy. Although this treatment was the major treatment of choice some one hundred years ago, today doctors may suggest its use especially if other surgical procedures or cryosurgery aren't successful in halting the progression of prostate cancer. In fact, Seymour C. Nash, M.D., who has served as chairman of the Urology Department at Mt. Sinai Hospital in Miami Beach, Florida, states that "in distant recurrence (meaning cancer metastasizing outside of the prostate gland) hormonal blockage is the prime and only choice of treatment." (Meyers, p. 212)

Side effects associated with the procedure are loss of sex drive (not in all cases), sterility, diarrhea, hot flashes (similar to hot flashes women encounter in menopause) and gynecomastia, (breast enlargement). Psychological and sociological problems often occur as men grapple with self-esteem issues following this procedure.

Radical Prostatectomy

The major goal of this surgery is to remove cancer localized within the prostate gland. The prostate gland is completely removed, as well as the seminal vesicle lines that secrete and store semen, the nerves to the penis and the lymph nodes.

In years past, in almost one hundred percent of cases this procedure meant impotency and the end of the ability to have an erection. Today, however, due to researchers at Johns Hopkins, a nerve-sparing procedure has been discovered that has reduced impotency rates to less than thirty percent. Other possible complications from this surgery are urinary incontinence, blood clots, pneumonia and even death.

Radiation Seed Implantation (Brachytherapy)

This procedure, also known as "internal radiation therapy," is carried out with the use of an ultrasound probe inserted into the rectum. An image of the prostate then appears on a television monitor. A radiation oncologist uses this visual image to guide the implantation of radioactive seeds into the prostate gland, inserting thin needles through the skin between the scrotum and the rectum.

After implantation, the radioactive seeds give off radiation for up to six months. This procedure allows more direct radiation to reach cells with minimal (if any) damage to healthy tissue. This procedure is tolerated well, especially by older patients who are unable to withstand the rigors of surgery.

Hormonal Drug Therapy

While the above therapies represent only a few of the most widely used treatments, medical professionals also employ a number of different drug therapies that are intended to reduce the production of androgens (male sex hormones). The drugs Flutamide and Leupron™ are commonly applied to inhibit the production of the testosterone that fuels the production of prostate cancer cells. Proscar™, the most widely prescribed drug used to treat symptoms related to BPH, as previously discussed, is used extensively.

The chart that follows gives a concise description of a few of the most popular drugs used today in the U.S. for the treatment of prostate disorders.

A plethora of drugs is used to treat BPH and inflammation of the prostate, as well as the bacterial and urinary tract infections

DRUGS USED TO TREAT PROSTATE DISORDERS

Medication (Common Name)	Medication Brand or Chemical Name	Mode of Action	How It Works	Side Effects
Proscar™	Finasteride	Hormonal	Slows down production of DHT (Shrinks prostate gland)	• impotency • decreased libido • reduced volume of semen
Hytrin™	Terazosin Hydrocholoride	Alpha Blocker	Causes muscles of prostate to relax, reducing pressure on urethra	• blurred vision • edema • drowsiness • fainting spells • weakness
Releasing Factor Antagonist Drugs Leupron™ Zolodex™	Releasing Factor Antagonist drug Leupron™ Zolodex™	Pituitary Gland	Signals pituitary gland at base of brain to stop production of testosterone	• loss of sex drive • hot flashes • heart disease
Eulexin™ Casodex™	Flutamide Bicalutamide	Hormonal	Blocks male hormone interaction with prostate cancer cells	• diarrhea • hot flashes • liver damage • loss of libido • impotence • nausea • gynecomastia (tenderness, pain or swelling of breast in men)
DES [a female hormone]	Diethystibesterl	Hormonal	Signals brain to stop production of testosterone by the testicles	• hot flashes • breast swelling • edema • blood clots • stroke

that often plague this gland. Commonly prescribed drugs include: amoxicillin, ampicillin, ceftizoxime, erythromycin, carbenicillin indanyl sodium and cipofloxacin.

ASK QUESTIONS AGAIN AND AGAIN

Before you and your doctor agree on a treatment plan, you should understand why one treatment is recommended over others. Evaluate the possible benefits, risks, side effects and impact on the quality of your life of the recommended treatment when compared with other treatments. The U.S. National Institute of Health has published a helpful brochure containing many of the questions that patients want to know about their treatment. (See: "When Cancer Recurs: Meeting the Challenge Again") The lists that follow are quoted from this publication. You may want to add your own questions to discuss with your doctor, nurse, or social worker. Family members or others close to you may have questions, too.

Questions to ask about any recommended treatment:

- What is the goal of this treatment? Is it a cure, will it shrink the tumor and relieve the symptoms, or is it for comfort only?
- Why do you think this treatment is the best one for me?
- Is this the standard treatment for my type of cancer?
- Are there other treatments? What are they?
- Am I eligible for any clinical trials?
- What benefits can I expect with this treatment? Are they temporary or permanent?
- Are there side effects with this treatment? Are they temporary or permanent?
- Is there any way to prevent or relieve the side effects?
- How safe is this treatment? What are the risks?
- Will I need to be in the hospital?
- What will happen if I don't have the treatment?

◆ What does my family need to know about the treatment? Can they help?
◆ How long will I be on this treatment?
◆ How much will the treatment cost?

About radiation therapy:

- What benefits can I expect from this therapy?
- What type of radiation treatment will I be getting?
- How long do the treatments take? How many will I need? How often?
- Can I schedule treatments at a certain time of day?
- What if I have to miss a treatment?
- What risks are involved?
- What side effects should I expect? What can I do about them?
- Who will give me the treatments? Where are they given?
- Will I need a special diet?
- Will my activities be limited?

About chemotherapy and hormone therapy:

- What do you expect the drugs to do for me?
- Which drugs will I be getting? How is each one given?
- Where are the treatments given?
- How long do the treatments take? How many will I need?
- What happens if I miss a dose?
- What risks are involved?
- What side effects should I expect? What can I do about them?
- Will I need a special diet or other restrictions?
- Can I take other medicines during treatment?
- Can I drink alcoholic beverages during treatment?

Before making an appointment with your doctor, review the questions above and write down any others you have. Remember, the decisions you make concerning treatment, especially in the case of cancer, have many quality-of-life issues attached to them. *It is your health and your life. If you don't understand an answer, ask another question until you do.*

In the next chapter we will take a look at some emerging alternative treatments that are gaining acceptance as viable options in treating disturbances of the prostate gland.

Please read on!

CHAPTER FIVE

ALTERNATIVE TREATMENTS

After years of denial, the National Cancer Institute has finally agreed with the vocal minority of nutritionists that diet is related to cancer, but they steadfastly deny the many successful alternative therapies which are available in various parts of the world.

—*Kurt W. Donsbach, D.C., N.D., Ph.D.*

As you would with any conventional treatment for prostate disturbance, it is just as important to discuss with your health practitioner the pros and cons of any alternative treatment, supplement or protocol. Your holistic medicine professional should do a work-up concerning your current status, and, depending on your individual case, order similar tests as would an allopathic (conventional medical) doctor. However, your holistic health practitioner will probably employ a number of natural, non-invasive programs to control and better manage associated symptoms and complications of BPH. Your treatment could consist of one or more of the following:

- ◆ Nutritional therapy
- ◆ Energy therapy
- ◆ Metabolic Mapping therapy
- ◆ Detoxification therapy

- Immune therapy
- Orthomolecular therapy
- Gene therapy
- Chelation therapy
- Ozone therapy
- Antioxidative therapies
- Herbal therapy
- Hydrotherapy
- Juice therapy
- Thymus therapy
- Guided Imagery therapy
- Weight Management therapies
- Hyperthermia
- Sound or Meditation therapy
- Antiangiogenesis therapy
- Photoluminescent therapy
- Colon therapy
- Biofeedback therapy
- Physiotherapy

Although many of these therapies may sound unfamiliar to you, they are commonplace practices used by alternative practitioners and in holistic health clinics and facilities throughout the U.S., in Europe, and around the world.

Despite the existence of successful alternatives, here in the United States there is a war being waged to maintain a one-dimensional healthcare system—a system in which treatments that have not been endorsed by the American Medical Association and similar organizations that fall under its umbrella, such as the National Cancer Institute or the American Cancer Society, are labeled as unproven. This is unwarranted, and in many cases downright negligent, according to Dr. Andrew Weil. One of the world's most notable experts in both medical and alternative modalities, Weil states that, "Allopathy as an organized enterprise is not only close-minded toward alternative practices but has waged constant and unfair war against other therapeutic systems, regarding them as competition rather than intellectual challenges." (1995, p. 119)

This defensive strategy of conventional medicine is being challenged, however, as we have cited earlier. The National Institute of Health (NIH) in the United States recently gave full status to the Office of Alternative Medicine, now called the National Center for Complementary and Alternative Medicine (NCCAM). This gives the center more authority and greater leeway in conducting research and overseeing the funding of research projects on the efficacy of alternative medicine. The center's budget went from $20 million in 1988 to $50 million in 1999.

We noted earlier that Dr. David Eisenberg of the Harvard School of Medicine found that in the U.S., visits to alternative medicine practitioners went from 427 million in 1990 to 629 million in 1997, actually exceeding total visits to all primary care physicians. In fact, a study conducted by researchers at the Health Policy Institute of the Medical College of Wisconsin, predicts a growth of rate of 124 percent in the number of alternative practitioners in the U.S. between 1994 and the year 2010, as compared to a sixteen percent growth rate in the number of conventional doctors.

Nonetheless, Dean King and Jonathan Pearlroth, authors of *Cancer Combat* and cancer survivors themselves, shared that when it came to fighting cancer via a more all-encompassing route, this often led them to unknown waters, meaning "unconventional treatments." Why, we ask, should an all-encompassing, health-rejuvenating program be viewed as "testing unknown waters"? (p. 249)

The answer seems to be that while conventional medicine focuses primarily on the use of drugs and surgery, alternative treatments aim at increasing the "functional ability" of the patient's natural disease-fighting mechanisms. Alternative practitioners view disorders of the prostate gland as "systemic disorders," meaning derangement of and consequent malfunction of normal metabolic patterns. It is because of the health-building and restorative benefits of alternative medicine modalities that people everywhere are now viewing them as viable options and using them in record numbers.

In the next section of this chapter we look at both emerging and standard alternative treatments for benign prostatic hyperplasia and prostate cancer. Many are and have been successfully used around the world.

Note: The listing or mention of a particular alternative protocol or treatment is not an endorsement by the author. They are listed and discussed for information purposes only. It is important that you discuss any treatment modality with your healthcare professional.

THE METHODS

Cholesterol Management

In addition to having patients who suffer from disorders of the prostate gland focus on weight management, alternative practitioners today place a strong emphasis on the management of proper cholesterol levels. When the body breaks down cholesterol, the waste by-products tend to find their way to and use worn, damaged or inflamed prostate tissue as a dumping ground. Invariably these metabolites of cholesterol cause healthy prostate cells to die. This can cause the prostate gland to enlarge. The bottom line here is to keep your cholesterol levels under 200 milligrams per deciliter of blood, to eliminate the use of highly saturated fats and to consume more flax, olive, soybean and sunflower oils.

Colon Therapy

To assist the colon in its efforts to remove toxins, alternative practitioners will suggest the use of acidophilus and FOS (fruitoglucosaccarides)—the good bacteria which reside in your intestinal tract. When this natural intestinal flora is compromised, unwanted harmful parasites can proliferate. This leaves the door open for an internal environment that encourages disease, including cancer, to develop.

In many cases holistic healthcare practitioners will suggest colonics. This procedure employs the use of large amounts of water to bathe the colon. It should only be administered by a qualified colon therapist. Additionally, the integration off fiber—25 to 50 grams introduced over several weeks in varying amounts, until the dose range is reached—is vital to maintaining good colon health. The slow introduction of fiber allows the system to adjust to this increased intake. Stomach cramps, pain, bloating and flatulence are common signs that too much fiber is being introduced too quickly.

Diet Therapy

The National Cancer Institute now concurs with nutritional advocates who have long claimed that there is a direct link between cancer and what we eat. The type of diet you consume can cause or accelerate the negative aspects of BPH. Processed foods, coffee, beer, soda, alcohol, and red peppers, to name a few, are all irritants to healthy prostate tissue. Red meat, saturated fats and cholesterol are natural born killers, so to speak, when it comes to the degeneration of the prostate gland. In fact, according to Dr. Edward A. Taub, founder of the Wellness Medicine Institute in Mt. Carmel, Illinois, and author of *The Wellness Rx*, men who eat red meat five times a week increase their chances of developing prostate cancer by 250 percent. (p. 41)

So, in the long and short of it, what you eat can go a long way in protecting you against the development of prostate disturbances. We shall cover the aspects of proper nutrition and its relationship to supporting good prostate health in Chapter Seven.

Detoxification

Detoxification is a much-used protocol because the prostate gland, as described previously, is a gland of vicarious elimination. When other glands of elimination such as the liver and the kidneys are overloaded with toxins, the body will use the prostate gland as a disposal site. For this reason it is vital that you keep your normal channels of elimination in good working order.

In cases of BPH, alternative practitioners will employ a number of protocols to insure that the need for vicarious elimination is reduced or eliminated. The goal of these programs is to increase the functionality of individual organs, as well as to create an internal environment that discourages the proliferation of cancerous cell growth.

The liver and gallbladder flush is a cornerstone of naturopathic detoxification routines. Refer to Appendix C in the back of this book for instructions on how to do this non-invasive natural treatment at home.

Note: Anyone currently suffering from gallbladder disease should consult a physician before undertaking the liver and gallbladder flush or another detoxification program.

Energy Medicine

This field is a vital part of the conceptual application of Chinese medicine. For ages the Chinese have professed that subtle levels of energy run through the body in neat patterns along pathways known as meridians. This fact has been recently validated by the National Institutes of Health's consensus statement on the efficacy of acupuncture. Acupuncturists use thin, solid, metallic needles to manipulate these energy meridians. According to a panel of medical experts in the U.S., China and Canada, in collaboration with the National Cancer Institute, the U.S. Office of Alternative Medicine, and the Office of Medical Applications Research in Bethesda, Maryland, there is sufficient evidence of acupuncture's potential value to conventional medicine to encourage further studies. (1997, p.19)

Rudolph Ballentine, M.D., director of The Center for Holistic Medicine in New York City and author of *Radical Healing,* states that "the subtle energetic aspect of human function is now becoming recognized as our technology becomes sophisticated and sensitive enough to measure it." (1999, p. 80) This energy, or *chi* (as it is called in Chinese medicine), is the internal force the body draws from to promote healing. Although this energy medicine is predicted to become the future of medicine in the new millennium, it is already common practice by many alternative practitioners in the U.S. and other countries around the world.

Many types of subtle energy treatment, such as ozone therapy, which are not allowed in the U.S., will be covered in more detail later in this chapter. When it comes to prostate disturbances, alternative practitioners will manipulate the body's natural energy or *chi* to improve blood flow to the gland, as well as to reduce oxidative stress. Oxidative stress refers to the formation of free radicals. Free radicals have been implicated in the development of up to sixty age-related diseases, including prostate cancer.

Supplements like CoQ10, Enada, vitamin E and vitamin C, as well as various detoxification programs, are used by alternative healthcare professionals to slow down free-radical aggression.

Presently, this invisible energy force is being called Tachyon energy in the U.S. According to Dr. Fouad I. Ghaly, former clinical professor of medicine at the University of Washington School of Medicine, the term "Tachyon energy" was first coined by Gerald Fienburg, Ph.D., a physicist at Columbia University in 1966. Deepak Chopra calls this life energy force "the invisible principle." Andrew Weil suggests that at its peak it may be the answer to the phenomenon of "spontaneous healing." (p. 130)

Exercise
While most of us are aware of the benefits of exercise and its relationship to cardiovascular health, fat burning and weight loss, it is now known that exercise contributes to good prostate health. As cited in a recent issue of *Nutritional Insights*, 12,975 men with an average age of forty-four were tracked for a nineteen-year period. Researchers found that consistent aerobic activity that burned off at least 3,000 calories a week decreased prostate cancer risk by seventy percent. (Burke, 1997)

Hydrotherapy
According to Michael Murray, N.D., the "sitz" bath is the number one form of hydrotherapy treatment used to treat an enlarged prostate gland. The sitz bath is usually administered by partial immersion of the pelvic region in a tub of alternating hot and cold water. The goal is to increase circulation to the muscles of the prostate gland and pelvic region, which helps relax and facilitate opening of the urinary passage.

Hyperthermia
In the past, fever was viewed as a negative factor. Alternative practitioners, however, view fever as a mechanism the body uses to kill foreign microbes, cancerous cells and other invaders. Widely used in Mexican hospitals and in Europe, the

use of controlled heat—called hyperthermia—is now being used to treat BPH and prostate cancer in the U.S. at Stanford University. Hyperthermia is generally used as an adjunct treatment to radiation and chemotherapy.

In this procedure, microwave heat at temperatures of 107° to 109.4° Fahrenheit is applied to the prostate gland. At these temperatures doctors have found that they can shrink an enlarged prostate gland and destroy cancerous tissue. In this procedure an instrument known as a Foley Catheter is inserted through the urethra. Cold water runs through this device to eliminate as much discomfort as possible.

While researchers aren't quite sure how hyperthermia actually works, it is believed that the heat relaxes the muscle tissue in the prostate, thus reducing the stronghold the prostate has on the urethra. This alleviates the obstructed flow of urine. This procedure in medical terms is called transurethral. Transrectal hyperthermia is the same procedure except that the catheter is inserted through the rectum. Treatments usually last about one hour. The transurethral procedure requires the use of a local anesthesia, while the transrectal does not. (Salmans, p. 112)

Immunotherapy

Kurt W. Donsbach, N.D., director of the Hospital Santa Monica in Rosarity Beach, Mexico, and Rudolf Alsleben, M.D., co-founder of the Health Restoration Institute in Tijuana, Mexico, report in their book, *Wholistic Cancer Therapy,* that cancer cells can disguise themselves from the body's natural immune system, which normally seeks out and destroys foreign or cancerous cells, bacteria and viruses. It is believed that cancer cells produce some sort of special chemical or use natural proteins found circulating in the blood to cover themselves, thereby tricking the immune system into thinking that these deadly predators are normal cells going about their daily duties, which is to produce metabolic energy to sustain life's processes.

The overall goal of immunotherapy is to stimulate the body's natural defense systems. Although this form of treatment dates back to the 1800s and is used widely in many alternative hospitals in Mexico, it is in the experimental stages in some of the major hospitals in the U.S.

Researchers maintain that more than one million lymphocytes (white blood cells) are armed and ready to prevent the development of cancer. The goal of the alternative physician is to enhance this inborn defense system. Depending upon the severity of your prostate problem, your practitioner may suggest one or a combination of the following to boost the workings of this internal defensive command post.

◆ Improving sleep patterns
◆ Fasting
◆ Change in dietary regimen
◆ Improving digestive functions
◆ Stopping or reducing smoking
◆ Colon therapy
◆ Reduction of stress
◆ Use of supplemental enzymes
◆ Detoxification
◆ Improving internal pH or homeostatic balance

Many of these approaches are covered in detail in this book. To find out more concerning these alternative modalities, and to connect with practitioners, websites and organizations that advocate them, refer to Chapter Nine, "Getting the Help You Need."

The Mind Factor

Many immune defenders are at work constantly waging a war on foreign matter entering the system. This battle goes on during our entire life cycle, every second of the day, because of the trillions of microorganisms in our system. There are invaders that work from within our systems as well as our own internal cells sometimes turn precancerous or change from their normal form. Dr. Lewis Thomas, former director of Memorial Sloan-Kettering Cancer Center, helped pioneer our understanding of how the mind and the immune system cooperate in their ability to defend us. This new and exciting field is called psychoneuroimmunology.

Dr. Carl Simonton, working with a technique called guided imagery, teaches his patients how to image the inner workings of their immune system fighting off invaders. Dr. Simonton has reported that some patients have envisioned knights on white horses, while others see tanks and fighter planes. At the Simonton Cancer Center in Pacific Palisades, California, visualization and mental imagery programs are designed to facilitate and enhance the other treatments a patient is already receiving.

Dr. Bernie S. Siegel, also a pioneer in mind/body medicine, likens our body and mind to an old dry, dusty basement. Siegel maintains that we tend to forget that our body stores our life's memories and experiences in every cell. He states, "the fact that we store memories in our bodies like we store old furniture in the basement should inspire us to start cleaning house, because leaving painful old memories can damage your residence [your body]." (p. 177)

Dr. Siegel's message is clear concerning our ability to control and manipulate our physical well-being via our own thought patterns. He adamantly claims that once we clean out the basement of negative thought patterns we will have more room to live.

While no one knows *how* mental images boost the immune response, researchers in this new and exciting field of mind/body medicine have reported dramatic results in combating disease, up to and including the shrinking of tumors in a number of cases. Joan Borysenko, Ph.D., a cell biologist, is one of the architects of this new field of psychoneuroimmunology. Dr. Borysenko is the former director of the mind/body clinic at New England Deaconess Hospital and the author of the *New York Times* bestseller, *Minding the Body, Mending the Mind.* Her work has personally helped thousands of patients enhance their physical well-being by using the mind as a weapon against disease.

Jon Kabat-Zinn, Ph.D., of the University of Massachusetts Medical Center in Worcester, has developed a clinical program based on meditation. Dr. Zinn finds that weak or deficient immune system responses can be enhanced by mastering simple meditation techniques. (Borysenko, 1993, pp. 164–166)

Because of the work of these pioneers and others, we now know that by improving our emotional and psychological state, we can not only prevent cancer and other maladies from occurring, but we also have an innate ability to cure them.

The Natural Prostate Massage

As we have learned, the prostate gland becomes a site for stubborn and reoccurring bacterial infections. Prostate massage gets a sluggish prostatic fluid moving. To massage the prostate gland, a doctor will insert a gloved finger into the patient's rectum.

The late Paavo Airola, N.D., an early pioneer of naturopathic medicine and an internationally recognized nutritionist, first introduced the concept of biological medicine to the United States in 1968. To naturally massage the prostate, Dr. Airola stressed the value of exercise, particularly in the form of walking. He also recommended the following as another form of exercise or natural massage for the prostate gland (1989, p. 143):

Step 1: Lie flat on your back.

Step 2: Pull the knees up as far as possible.

Step 3: Press the soles of both feet together.

Step 4: Holding the soles pressed together, lower the legs as far as possible with forceful repeated movements. Repeat several times.

Note: I advise the use of this simple exercise as a preventive measure to be done one to three times a week. However, as with any exercise routine, it is important to check with your healthcare professional before starting.

Don't Forget to Kegel

In the 1950s, Dr. Arnold Kegel, a gynecologist, introduced a simple exercise (now known as "Kegels") to help women regain bladder control after childbirth. Over the years, Kegels have been found to be of great benefit to men with continence difficulties, and as a means of naturally massaging the prostate gland.

For a moment, tighten or clench the muscle in your groin that you would use to stop the flow of urine when urinating; the same muscle you would use to force out the last drop of urine from your bladder. This is called the PC or pubococcygeal muscle. Each time you tighten and then release that muscle you are doing a Kegel exercise.

Starting today, I recommend that you make Kegels a part of your daily routine for prostate health. To begin:

1. Clench and relax the PC muscle repeatedly (about ten times in succession), but slowly, holding the tension for three to five seconds each time, then releasing it.

2. Do the above sequence five times a day.

3. Gradually work toward doing the exercises thirty times in succession, holding for three to five seconds each time. Repeat this procedure three times a day.

According to Dr. Kenneth Goldberg, medical director of the Male Health Institute, Baylor Health Center, Irving-Coppell, Texas and editor of the *Men's Health Book,* it will take about four to six weeks to get your PC muscle in good shape. When you do, you will be better able to control incontinence problems related to prostate disturbances.

An added plus to the practice of Kegel exercises is that of sexual gratification and the elimination of stagnation of excess prostatic fluid. The PC muscle that helps to control urine flow is also responsible for the force of ejaculation. By mastering Kegels you can make your erection firmer and magnify the intensity of the release of prostatic fluids and your orgasms. So, don't forget to Kegel daily!

Urinary Tract Detoxification
When the urinary tract becomes too alkaline, it invites bacterial growth. Some alternative healthcare doctors will recommend that you decrease the pH content of the system. Eating more whole-grain cereal products, cottage cheese and other

natural cheeses, and animal protein for a week or so will decrease the pH and raise the body's acidic nature.

"Potential of hydrogen," commonly referred to as pH, is a measure of the alkalinity or acidity of the body's internal environment on a scale of 1 to 14. A reading is made from a test strip that has been dipped in the patient's urine sample. A reading from 1 to 6 indicates the body is acidic. Seven is neutral, while 8 to 14 is alkaline.

Nutritionally manipulating this internal environment toward the acidic side will help the body stop unwanted bacterial growth in the urinary tract. This treatment should only be employed during acute episodes of infection and shouldn't be considered a part of a regular daily dietary regimen.

Drinking two to four glasses of cranberry juice daily is very helpful for natural detoxification, as cranberry juice discourages the growth of harmful bacteria in the urinary tract.

I employ the use of the following detoxification routine to assist in keeping my urinary tract in good health. For a two-week period, every other month, with each meal I drink an eight-ounce glass of water mixed with two tablespoons of apple cider vinegar and one tablespoon of natural honey.

Weight Loss

One of the best things you can do to protect yourself from the negative effects of prostate disturbances is to lose that extra weight. Researchers now know that men who are overweight are two-and-a-half times more likely than men of normal weight to develop prostate cancer. Alternative practitioners advocate programs to increase the muscle-to-fat ratio. The high metabolic capacity of muscle will help the body burn up calories much faster, thus encouraging a lean and trim body. This is paramount for maintaining good prostate health. As a point of reference, an acceptable body fat range of twelve to eighteen percent is considered good for males.

Researchers at Beijing Medical University in China validated the association of weight gain and faltering prostate functions in studies conducted as early 1977. (Gu, pp. 163–166)

Metabolic Balancing

Rather than treating individual symptoms of illness, or separate body organs or "parts," one of the cornerstones of alternative medicine is identifying and making adjustments to a patient's lifestyle and habits to create a balanced metabolism of the body as a whole. Alternative practitioners tend to view disease as systemic—meaning that disease is a manifestation of multiple health problems.

The body goes through diverse patterns of metabolic activity in its attempts to reduce and rebuild tissue. These frenzied, but precisely controlled and beneficial events, when severely out of balance, have been linked to prostate disturbances and other degenerative diseases. Dr. Tom Spies, who served as a professor of nutrition and metabolism at Northwestern Medical School, continuously expressed need to look at the whole picture:

> Germs are no longer our principle enemy. Our greatest emerging medical problem is the disturbance of the inner balance of the constituents of our tissues that are built from and maintained by necessary chemicals in the air we breath, the water we drink and the food we eat. (Cheraskin et.al., 1987, p. 7)

Such imbalance can lead to depressed immunity, accelerated cancer growth and an internal environment that encourages degeneration. Metabolic balancing, as practiced by many alternative practitioners, attempts to remedy this. These doctors will focus on increasing the strength of all your internal organs and systems, thereby assisting the normal metabolic efficiency of the body.

Metabolic balancing may consist of correcting faulty or insufficient digestive patterns and lack of natural energy reserves, enhancing the body's detoxification and elimination capabilities, and increasing the body's ability to defend itself from free-radical aggression, thus protecting the cells and their precious cargo, DNA.

One company at the forefront of assessing blood and chemical metabolic interrelationships is the Human Technologies Group of Greenbrae, California. To find out more about having a metabolic profile done, call, or have your healthcare practitioner contact, Linda Alber, Health-Map Technologies, 405 Via Casitas, Suite 1, Greenbrae, California 94904, (415-464-1200.)

TAKING A LOOK AROUND THE WORLD

We will now examine some treatments that have been used extensively outside the U.S. Due to the limits imposed by the United States Food and Drug Administration, certain treatment protocols are illegal in the U.S. For example, the administration of the Gerson Therapy, a complex diet plan that emphasizes drinking large amounts of freshly-prepared vegetable juices to treat cancer, is against the law. The use of ozone, laetrile (from apricot pits), live cell therapy, hydrogen peroxide therapy, magnetic energy therapy and gene therapy are considered "unproven treatments" by the traditional U.S. medical community.

However, according to Dr. Kurt Donsbach, director of the Hospital Santa Monica in Rosarito Beach, Mexico, "the treatments and medicines most often used by the alternative practitioner are not concocted in his bathtub, but instead are often commonplace in other parts of the world." (p.1) Donsbach states that at the Hospital Santa Monica they use "17 non-toxic remedies which have over 1,000 medical references to justify their use and effectiveness."

In a related matter, Jane Heimlich, the wife of the doctor who developed the Heimlich maneuver to prevent choking, in her book *What Your Doctor Won't Tell You,* cites an article in *American Medical News* (August 9, 1985) titled "Unorthodox Clinics Flourishing in Tijuana." (p. 281) This piece focused on the astonishing survival rates of patients with prostate and other cancers. People often come to these Mexican hospitals after conventional approaches have failed, and when they have been told there is nothing more that can be done.

Dominican Republic

One of the emerging treatment protocols that is causing quite a stir in the Dominican Republic is called "cell specific cancer therapy." This technique, which is being pioneered at the Center for Cell Specific Cancer Therapy in Santa Domingo, uses magnetic energy generated from a donut-shaped ring or collar composed of magnets. The device, called a CSCT-200, emits an electromagnetic current. This electromagnetic field can be manipulated to target only cancer cells, destroying them without harming healthy cells. There are no side effects reported, nor delayed reactions to contend with.

To date, fifty percent of the patients treated since the Center's opening in 1996 have had successful remissions of various cancers. Opponents of this therapy contend that the long-term success rate cannot be addressed due to the short time frame of the Center's existence.

Seoul, Korea and Tijuana, Mexico

Rodrigo Rodriguez, M.D., of the American Biologic Hospital, Tijuana, Mexico, and Woo-chul Moon, M.D., Ph.D., professor at the Chung-Ang University Hospital in Seoul, Korea, are pioneering the use of a program called "p53 gene therapy." Used to treat advanced stages of prostate, rectum, bladder, and other types of cancer, this treatment focuses on tumor suppression and angiogenesis (the formation of new blood vessels) destruction. According to these researchers, when p53 DNA is introduced into the body of a cancer patient, "cancer cells die, stop growing and do not metastasize to other parts of the body." (p. 3)

In fact, Dr. Rodriguez and Dr. Moon claim that most of the chemotherapy drugs used by oncologists do not actually kill cancer cells. Rather, the job of these drugs is to activate p53, which kills cancer cells.

While this treatment is not part of treatment protocols in the U.S., information cited in the National Cancer Institute's handbook, *Understanding Gene Testing,* does define the role of tumor suppressor genes as genes that normally restrain cell growth, but, when missing or inactivated by mutation, allow cells to grow uncontrolled. (1995, p. 30)

Germany

Carnivora is a natural substance extracted from the *Dionea muscipula* plant, commonly known as the venus flytrap. The ability of this natural substance to combat prostate cancer has been advocated by Dr. Morton Walker, U.S. medical and nutritional researcher. Based on his research years ago, Dr. Walker suggested that President Ronald Reagan and the actor Yul Brenner include this natural substance as part of their battle plan against cancer.

Carnivora was first researched and discovered in 1971 by Dr. Helmut Keller of the Department of Oncology at the Tumor Clinic in Obersatufen, Germany. Dr. Keller began testing the effects of *carnivora* more extensively at Boston University in the U.S. in 1973. He found that a potent nontoxic chemical called "plumbagin" in *carnivora* was responsible for its ability to fight cancer by producing superoxidizers and hydrogen peroxide, naturally. Plumbagin also accelerates the production of more active killer T-cells, the body's anticancer patrol force. Today, Dr. Keller treats patients at his clinic in Bad Steben, Germany.

Also, German researchers were the first to conduct human trials on the efficacy of the plant extracts from the herb *Serenoa repens,* commonly known as saw palmetto. German scientists had discovered that substances known as plant sterols in *serenoa repens* had the ability to block or slow down the negative effects of 5-alpha-reductase, the enzyme responsible for converting DHT (dihydrotestosterone) into testosterone. As we learned earlier, it is this conversion that accelerates the production of cancerous prostate cells.

In New Zealand and Saudi Arabia, saw palmetto in known as Permixon. We will review this natural supplement in more detail in Chapter Six.

Greece

In the early 1950s, Dr. Evangelos Danopoulos of the Medical School of Athens University discovered that urea could control or slow down the growth of cancerous cells. (Urea is a waste by-product of protein digestion and is normally eliminated when you urinate.) Dr. Danopoulos discovered that a mixture in solution of fifty percent urea that was extracted, purified and isolated had the ability to inhibit tumor growth. As reported in the *Alternative Medicine Digest* (Issue 17, 1997, p. 69), when

Danopoulos injected this solution around the tumor cite it interrupted the process that hastens uncontrolled cell growth.

India

The oldest system of healing known to humankind is that of
ayurveda. Ayurveda, which means "the science of life," is a
6,000-year-old system of healing which has its origin in India.
Through the teachings of Dr. Deepak Chopra this ancient system is gaining acceptance in the U.S.

Vasant Lad, B.A.M.S., M.A.Sc., a native of India and one of
only a handful of classically-trained ayurvedic doctors teaching in the U.S., is credited with bringing much of what is known
about this healing system to the Western world.

One natural supplement used by ayurvedic practitioners to
purify the blood as well as to boost the body's natural immunity
is *manjistha*. This botanical (herb) is touted for its ability to assist the body's natural ability to destroy toxins in the blood, and
also to increase blood flow and inhibit blood stagnation. This
property of *manjistha* could contribute to good prostate health,
as toxins have a way of finding their way to the prostate gland,
thus accelerating oxidative reactions with free radicals.

Japan

It is no secret that Japanese men suffer far less than American
men from disorders of the prostate gland. Researchers contend
that this fact is primarily due to the Japanese diet, which consists of very little red meat, saturated fat and processed food.
What do Japanese men eat? Lots of vegetables (including sea
vegetables), soy products and generous amounts of fish. Besides the powerful antioxidant properties of these food products, they also have anti-angiogenesis properties. Substances
that are classified as having anti-angiogenetic properties can
assist in the destruction of cancer cells by inhibiting the growth
of new blood vessels, which are the lifeline of the cancerous
cell or tumor.

The Japanese also have the distinction of having discovered
a non-toxic natural substance which is the most widely used

in the world to treat various types of cancer. This product is known as Krestin. Krestin is a polysaccharide complex carbohydrate or starch formed from strings of glucose units of a Japanese mushroom. Researchers at Hokkaido University School of Medicine in Sapporo, Japan, discovered that Krestin and lentinan, another chemical compound found in mushrooms, increased depressed immunity and enhanced killer T-cell activity in lab animals with cancer. Administered orally, Krestin has been found to be effective in tumor reduction of a number of different cancers when combined with standard drugs such as mitomycin-C, an antibiotic.

The Japanese are credited with introducing the macrobiotic diet to the Western world. The diet consists of fifty percent whole grain cereals, twenty to thirty percent organically-grown vegetables, plus small portions of soups, beans, fish and sea vegetables. Michio Kushi has presented evidence of this diet's ability to prevent as well as restore health when cancer is present in his book, *The Cancer Prevention Diet* (1983).

In a subsequent chapter we will take a look at the macrobiotic diet and its role in one U.S. medical doctor's triumph over prostate cancer.

Mexico

Oxygen therapy is one of the treatments employed by Dr. Donsbach to slow the destructive nature of prostate and other cancers. The theory behind this treatment is centered on the fact that cancer flourishes in an anaerobic environment. Cancer cells can't proliferate in an environment in which oxygen is active in live tissue, as oxygen inhibits cancer's ability to survive and grow.

Oxygen is administered in several ways: intravenously via hydrogen peroxide, orally via hydrogen peroxide, through hydrogen peroxide and ozone baths, and by ozone (a form of oxygen) insufflation. (p. 6) This infusion of fresh oxygen to the cells revitalizes normal tissue while suffocating cancerous tissue.

Gerard V. Sunken, M.D., an associate professor at New York University, has been trying to get ozone therapy approved in the U.S. since 1985. Despite at least fifty-nine references on positive clinical reports and animal studies using ozone therapy, this therapy is still classified as unproven in the U.S., according to Dr. Sunken. (Heimlich, 1990)

In 1983, the Gerson Institute started inclusion of this therapy in its programs. Ozone therapy is utilized throughout Europe and at other alternative health clinics in Mexico as well.

The Gerson Therapy

The Gerson Therapy was first developed and introduced by Dr. Max Gerson, a German physician (1881–1959). Dr. Gerson's treatment protocols have now been in existence for over sixty years and are utilized worldwide. The Gerson Institute, located in Bonita, California, offers instructions to both alternative and conventional healthcare professionals, as well as to individuals wishing to incorporate the Gerson Therapy into their daily lives. Oasis of Hope, located in Tijuana, Mexico, just thirty minutes from San Diego, California, is the only fully-accredited hospital in North America licensed by the Gerson Institute. Licensing in this context refers to the hospital's ability to administer the full and complete Gerson Therapy as a cancer treatment.

The Gerson Therapy is centered on the detoxification of the body and the restorative capabilities of the body's natural healing power. In essence, the goal of this therapy is to restore the body's metabolic potential, thus fostering an internal environment that is not conducive for prostate cancer, or any cancer, to flourish.

During the course of this therapy the body is flooded with the juice of up to twenty pounds of organically-grown fruits and vegetables daily. One glass of fresh juice every hour, or thirteen times a day, is consumed. The therapy also incorporates a nutritional program that includes:

- ◆ a low-fat diet with little animal protein
- ◆ a high carbohydrate diet (fruit, organic vegetables and grains)
- ◆ a low sodium to high potassium ratio
- ◆ the use of supplemental potassium

According to Ralph W. Moss, Ph.D., the author of *Cancer Therapy*, a Pulitzer Prize nominee, and former Assistant Director of Public Affairs at the Memorial Sloan-Kettering Cancer Center, long-term studies of the Gerson Therapy have been conducted by Dr. Peter Lechner of Graz, Austria. From his research, Dr. Lechner concluded that the Gerson Therapy in most cases can deter, slow down and prevent "cachexia." Cachexia is the wasting away that occurs with prostate and other cancer patients. (p. 192)

Overall, this therapeutic protocol may assist in making the patient functionally stronger. We will cover the importance of dietary factors in more detail in Chapter Seven.

Oasis of Hope offers a full line of alternative medical treatments to fight disorders of the prostate gland. Many of these treatments—including laetrile usage—are not standard treatments in the United States. (For more information call 1-888-500-HOPE.)

Sweden

Since the early 1930s and 1940s, reports out of Sweden describe a natural product made from flower pollen and its ability to reduce the severity of prostatitis. Today this product is marketed under the name Cernitin, and is sold over the counter in health stores in the United States. This naturally occurring product is widely used in Europe, Malaysia, Hong Kong, Japan and Taiwan.

Recent studies conducted on the effectiveness of Cernitin at the Department of Urology at Kyoto University, Japan, revealed that 41.7 percent of the patients studied reported the product as being effective in controlling symptoms associated with BPH, while an additional 41.7 percent reported Cernitin to be slightly effective. Only sixteen percent reported it to be ineffective. This product works by relaxing the muscles of the bladder and prostate gland, helping to improve urine flow.

Harry G. Preuss M.D., professor at Georgetown University Medical Center and a member of the Advisory Council for the Office of Alternative Medicine at the U.S. National Institute of Health, states that the results of this study are significant. Yet, the fact is that while Cernitin has been widely researched and is now used in nearly every country in the world, it is virtually unknown in the United States. (p. 102)

The Bahamas

While there has been and continues to be ongoing research concerning immunology and the enhancement of this inborn system of defense, the practice of "immune augmentative therapy" is not approved for use in the U.S. Formulated by Lawrence Burton, Ph.D., a zoologist, the treatment involves administering a blood serum made from human proteins. According to Dr. Burton, prostate cancer patients have had great success with this serum administered at his clinic in the Bahamas.

Since no formal research papers or scientific studies validating Dr. Burton's claims have been presented, researchers from other countries, including the U.S., have been unable to substantiate his claims.

IN CONCLUSION

As a holistic health practitioner, teacher and researcher, the most important thing to me is that I am still learning. There is, however, one question that continues to surface with regard to every new natural supplement, protocol or treatment modality I come across. *If around the globe many of these so-called alternative or unproven treatments or modalities are commonplace, and many of these countries rank much higher than the United States in the overall health of their citizens, why don't these non-surgical methods warrant extensive investigation here in the U.S.?*

It is my belief that as alternative medicine is further integrated into mainstream medicine (meaning allopathic medicine), it will not receive the attention to detail and continued expansion and research the public wants here in the U.S. This is unfortunate, since each year the U.S. spends more to treat illness and disease than virtually all the other nations of the world put together, states Edward Taub, M.D. (p. 3)

PART THREE

Supplements and Foods for Prostate Health

Many allopathic patients are surprised to learn of the existence of wholly drugless systems of treatment.

—*Andrew Weil, M.D.*

CHAPTER SIX

NATURAL–BORN MEDICAMENTS

> There is a nutrient or nutrients for nearly every drug that accomplishes the same function in the body.
>
> —*Sherry A. Rogers, M.D.*

Is it true that there may be a natural supplement more effective than your drug? According to Michael T. Murray, N.D., author of *Natural Alternatives to Over-the-Counter and Prescription Drugs,* most likely the answer is yes. (p. 35) This train of thought coincides with that of Dr. Sherry Rogers, cited above. A specialist in environmental medicine, Dr. Rogers has lectured in medical schools and colleges in over fifty U.S. cities and in six countries. Rogers, who has been in private practice in Syracuse, New York, for over twenty-six years, is one of the new breed of doctors who focuses on the medical application of nutrition and supplementation to fight many of today's chronic disorders, including prostate disturbances.

Although many patients in allopathic treatment are still unaware of the benefits of natural supplements as viable options to drugs, this trend is changing worldwide. For example, in the United States, the National Center for Complementary and Alternative Medicine is now a fully functional government agency with the sole purpose of conducting research into the safety and medicinal value of herbs and other nutritional supplements. In Canada, the government is setting aside $6.6 million to establish a federal office to evaluate and regulate botanicals (herbal medicines), as well as other alternative products. In Germany, the German Commission E sets many of the worldwide standards on the use and production of herbal products. In Mexico, sales of natural supplements totaled $360 million in 1998.

Sales of natural supplements have skyrocketed in the U.S. over the last decade. The U.S. is the largest nutritional market in the world according to a recent study published by the *Nutrition Business Journal*. In 1997, consumer sales of dietary supplements and organic foods reached $23 billion dollars. Data show that global sales of dietary supplements and organic foods in 1997 totaled $65 billion.

A study released in June of 1999 by the *Nutrition Business Journal* revealed that sales of natural supplements via the Internet had reached $40 million in 1998. This was an increase of twelve million dollars in one year: going from $28 million in 1997 to $40 million in 1998. It is estimated that Internet sales of natural products will reach $160 million by the end of 1999, with projected Internet sales of $500 million annually by the year 2001. (*Vitamin Retailer*, 1999, p.18)

The focus of this chapter is to introduce you to natural supplements and products once considered unapproved, or as "underground" entities. Many of these supplements are, however, currently being viewed as viable options to drugs in treating conditions related to benign prostatic hyperplasia.

Although the scope of this book does not permit covering all the natural supplements currently being used, we will cover many of the most popular. To assess the overall effectiveness of these natural alternatives the chapter is divided into eight short sections, each section covering one category of natural supplements or products—amino acids, antioxidants, enzymes, herbs, hormones, accessory supplements, vitamins and minerals, and whole food factors.

AMINO ACIDS

Amino acids are known as the building blocks of protein. Their health-restoring benefits have received much attention over the last decade. The body uses amino acids to rebuild new tissue structures for virtually all its growth and repair needs, including that of the prostate gland. There are currently twenty-two known amino acids; eight of them are called essential, meaning that the body is incapable of making them, so they have to be supplied by dietary or supplemental means.

Interest in amino acids stems from the fact that many of them are sulfur-bearing and thus protect the prostate gland and the liver. The amino acids glycine, alanine and glutomine can improve complications associated with BPH. Alan L. Miller, N.D., cites a study of forty-five men, of whom one-half were given 390 combined milligrams of these three amino acids three times a day for two weeks, then one capsule once daily for an additional week. The other half were given a placebo. At the end of this trial, as reported in *Alternative Medicine Digest* (Aug/Sept 1998, p. 14):

◆ Sixty-six percent of the amino acid group had less urinary urgency, and

◆ Fifty percent reported less difficulty urinating.

The amino acid glutamine, used in hospitals to help prevent muscle wasting, is beneficial in supporting good prostate function. Glutamine is the primary fuel used by the body to run immune system activities. It is a well-known fact that in human physiology the majority of the energy supplied to the cells is in the form of glucose. However, the immune system uses glutamine as its primary source of fuel. The major problem with maintaining adequate glutamine levels—about 120 grams, which the body naturally produces—is that illness depletes it. During periods of chronic stress, inflammation, pain and episodes of suppressed immune function, glutamine supplementation is warranted.

Note: If you begin a daily regimen of amino acid supplementation, use a naturally-occurring formula that contains a full complement of all the amino acids. Also make sure that your aminos are listed on the product label as being in their "L-forms" and not DL forms. L-forms are natural and are biologically ready to interact with human tissue. Your prostate gland will thank you for it.

ANTIOXIDANTS

Antioxidants are considered one of the most important medical discoveries in the last fifty years. They protect the body against free radicals. Free radicals are highly reactive molecules that have been implicated as the cause of over sixty age-related degenerative diseases, such as prostate cancer. For individuals suffering from disorders of the prostate gland, antioxidant support is critical.

Grape Seed Extract

This antioxidant, used extensively in France, is vital for assisting with circulation and maintaining the integrity of capillaries, the small blood vessels that form the foundation of the cardiovascular system. Scientists have discovered that the active ingredient found in grape seed extract—proanthocyanidins—is responsible for its dynamic capabilities. Besides immobilizing free-radical aggression, proanthocyanidins have the ability to destroy cancerous cells.

The antioxidant capability of grape seed extract has been described as being ten to twenty times greater than that of vitamin C and vitamin E.

From a prevention standpoint, the use of grape seed extract to shield the prostate from oxidative stress caused by free radicals will go a long way toward supporting proper prostate function.

IP-6™

IP-6™ is one of the new and exciting natural substances used to limit the internal destruction caused by free radicals. It has gained national attention due to its ability to help prevent and treat cancer. Backed by extensive scientific research conducted mainly by Abulkalam M. Shamsuddin, M.D., Ph.D., professor of pathology at the University of Maryland School of Medicine in Baltimore, IP-6™—short for inositol hexaphosphate—is a natural substance found in whole grains such as rice, oats, wheat and corn, plus beans, citrus fruits, pork, and nuts. Current research has revealed that IP-6™:

◆ Accelerates natural killer cell activity

◆ Slows down the rate of cancer cell division

◆ Can prevent free-radical aggression

◆ Can normalize cancer cells

According to Dr. Shamsuddin, this activity is vital to the prevention and treatment of any type of cancer, since cancer is essentially a disease of replication. IP-6™ can be purchased in health and vitamin stores as the product called Cell Forte with IP-6™, marketed by Enzymatic Therapy. (You can call Enzymatic Therapy at 1-800-783-2286.) According to Dr. Shamsuddin, IP-6™ should be taken in these dose ranges:

◆ To maintain normal health, 1 to 2 grams per day

◆ For persons with a high risk of developing cancer, 2 to 4 grams daily

IP-6™ is best taken on an empty stomach in between meals to enhance absorption. Make sure when purchasing IP-6™ that the formulation includes the B vitamin inositol. Inositol greatly enhances the overall effectiveness of IP-6™.

Lipoic Acid

Lipoic acid has been the subject of extensive study over the last decade because of its ability to help keep blood glucose levels stabilized. Today, lipoic acid is used by alternative medical practitioners to assist in the management of diabetes. Researchers also have learned that lipoic acid has powerful antioxidant capabilities itself, while simultaneously being able to regenerate other antioxidants—much like jump-starting a car battery that has lost some of its power.

One of the major advantages with the use of lipoic acid is that it works as both a water-soluble and fat-soluble nutrient. In other words, lipoic acid has no limitations within human physiology, and as such is known as a whole-body metabolic enhancer.

For superior antioxidant protection I highly recommend its use. Current data indicate that for optimal antioxidant protection lipoic acids should be taken in dosages of 100 mg three times a day.

Soy

Unless you have been keeping company with Rip Van Winkle for the last few years, I'm sure you've heard or have been told about the benefits of soy. Ironically, this information may have come from your spouse, or a female co-worker or acquaintance concerned about breast cancer.

Soy contains a powerful antioxidant called genisten. Dr. Harry Preuss, at Georgetown University Medical Center, states that "genisten has estrogen-like properties, which may inhibit the growth of prostatic cancer in its early development." (1998, p.144) Additionally, researchers like Derrick M. DeSilva, Jr., M.D., president of the American Nutraceutical Association and director of the Raritan Bay Medical Center in Perth Amboy, New Jersey, claim that soy, called soy isoflavonoids in supplement form, inhibits the process of angiogenesis, the pathological process in which cancer cells form new blood vessels to nourish themselves. (pp. 14-15)

The bottom line here is that soy powder, soy foods and soy supplements are not just for women as a preventive measure against breast cancer. Men too should be eating soy products as a means of preventing prostate cancer.

Dr. Walter Troll, professor of Environmental Science at New York University Medical Center, theorizes that if everyone consumed more soy-based products and soybeans, they could lessen the severity of cancer, but more importantly prevent it in the first place. (*Natural Pharmacy News*, 1999, p. 8)

Suggested Dose:

- 100 to 160 grams of soy-based food daily. This would equal about 4–8 ounces.

- In supplement form (soy isoflavonoids), 10 to 15 mg three times a day

ENZYMES

Controversy exists concerning the role of enzymes and their use to treat symptoms associated with BPH. Since disorders of the prostate gland are considered to be systemic in nature, researchers have found that enzymes assist in normalizing metabolic processes. Enzymes are actually the body's labor force. They could be compared to the mainframe of a central computer, responsible for the proficient minute-to-minute operation of the network connected to it.

In human systems the enzymes keep the "mainframe" operating—in this case the human body. Without enzymes we are essentially a conglomeration of chemicals unable to function. Well-known physicians like Robert Atkins and Joseph Weissman, a board-certified immunologist and assistant clinical professor at the University of California Medical School, employ the use of supplemental enzymes in their practices. Dr. Weissman states that "staying healthy may be relative to the amount of enzymes in our bodies." (Weiner, 1996, p. 4)

Dr. Atkins routinely uses enzymes at his clinic to fight malignancies. In reference to preventing and treating prostate dysfunction, the goal is not to enhance digestion (although this is an added benefit), but to eat away fibrin shields. Fibrin is a strong, white, elastic fibrous protein.

As we have learned, prostate problems can take decades to develop. It is now known that cancer cells have a way of making themselves appear normal, thus avoiding an all-out assault by the immune system. Enzymes destroy the fibrin shields that prostate cancer cells and other cancerous cells hide in. In addition, enzymes help reduce inflammation that often occurs within the prostate gland.

Although under ideal conditions the pancreas pumps out about half a gallon of solution filled with enzymes, I strongly suggest that you incorporate the use of a multiple enzyme formula into your daily supplement protocol. Because there is a strong correlation between aging and disorders of the prostate gland, our overall production of enzymes—these tireless workers—diminishes with age. In fact, a sixty-year-old could have fifty percent fewer enzymes than a thirty-year-old. Without enzymes operating at fully capacity, the body must deal with an environment conducive to causing prostate dysfunction.

Note: Due to the extensive research done with enzymes in Germany, I highly recommend the use of a product called Wobenzymes. They are available in vitamin and health stores here in the U.S. Enzymatic Therapy also has a very good formula called Mega-zyme, also found in vitamin and health food stores.

HERBS

Herbs have been valued since the beginning of time for their medicinal properties. Many of the drugs manufactured today originate from herbal sources. Herbal remedies in their whole or unadulterated state are gaining in popularity around the globe as viable options to synthetic drugs.

Essiac®

This herbal remedy has a long history of use as a potent anti-cancer agent and immune system modulator. It also is a powerful detoxifier and blood cleanser. Formulated in 1922 by the late Rene Caisse (Essiac® is Caisse spelled backward), a Canadian nurse, this herbal combo is used today mainly in tea form. Dr. Julian Whitaker strongly recommends that anyone suffering from cancer, including prostate cancer, begin incorporating

Essiac® tea into their existing regime. Dr. Whitaker suggests (1995, p. 4):

1. If you have cancer, drink two fluid ounces three times a day for twelve consecutive weeks without interruption.
2. For its overall health-promoting ability, two cups should be consumed twice a day for two weeks. Then one cup daily for maintenance.

Note: For overall health the above process can be done daily for fourteen days, then repeated in two weeks.

Essiac® combines the health restorative power of four herbs: burdock root, slippery elm, turkey rhubarb and sheep sorrell. Essiac® also contains inulin, a very potent immune system regulator. Inulin works by connecting to the surface of white blood cells, known as T-cells, thus enhancing their immune and anti-cancer capabilities.

Garlic

This herb has a 5000-year history of use. In China, garlic is used to treat dysentery (infection of the colon) and intestinal parasites. Dubbed "nature's natural antibiotic," garlic's anti-cancer and medicinal properties are attributed to its naturally-occurring sulfur compounds. These compounds protect the prostate and other internal systems and glands against free-radical damage.

Garlic's properties were recently confirmed by researchers at the Memorial Sloan-Kettering Cancer Center. Richard S. Rivlin, director of Clinical Nutrition at Sloan, reported in *Science News* (Vol. 51, April 19, 1997) that prostate cancer cells exposed to S-allymercaptocysteine (sam-C), a sulfur compound formed when garlic ages, caused cancer cells to break down testosterone much more rapidly. The researchers concluded from their research that sam-C was essentially performing the same function as treatments designed to slow down the conversion of DHT to testosterone.

An added benefit is the ability of aged garlic extract to modulate glutathione activity. Glutathione is one of the most potent liver detoxifiers used to support immunity.

Nettles

This herb, also known as stinging nettles, is used to support good prostate health by reducing inflammation of the prostate gland.

PC Spes

This formula, whose name invokes a vision of a character out of a James Bond movie, is a new product that is showing great promise. PC Spes is a synergistic formula that contains a combination of Chinese herbs revered for their ability to modulate immune function, as well as to support and enhance the functions of your hormonal systems. This herbal formula is composed of the following herbs traditionally used in Chinese medicine:

- ◆ Chrysanthemum (detoxifier)
- ◆ Licorice (anti-inflammatory)
- ◆ Ganoderma lucidum (a mushroom immune stimulant)
- ◆ Rubescent (immune stimulation)
- ◆ Ginseng (adaptogen stress relief)
- ◆ Saw Palmetto (hormonal balance)
- ◆ Isatis indigotica (antibacterial agent)
- ◆ Scutellania bacicalensis (detoxifier)

PC Spes, when administered orally in dose ranges of 2,700 mgs daily, caused PSA levels to drop dramatically, according to James Lewis, Ph.D., and E. Roy Berger, M.D., authors of *New Guidelines for Surviving Prostate Cancer.* For example, a patient fifty-two years of age went from a PSA of 40 to 20 after four weeks on PC Spes. According to Dr. Lewis, also author of *How I Survived Prostate Cancer* and executive director of The Education Center for Prostate Cancer Patients (a national non-profit organization) located in New York, PC Specs shows great promise. Lewis and Berger, a medical oncologist whose chief field of expertise is prostate cancer, recount the case of a seventy-four-year-old patient whose PSA score after using PC Spes went from 136 to 61—this after forty-two months of prior conventional treatment.

Both Dr. Berger and Dr. Lewis maintain that PC Spes could possibly be used as an adjunct to hormonal therapy. According to Lewis, ninety percent of all men taking drugs to control secretions of sex hormones (testosterone or estrogen) eventually reach a plateau, medically known as "hormonal refractive disease," when the body builds a tolerance to these drugs.

Note: For more information about PC Spes refer to *New Guidelines for Surviving Prostate Cancer* (Westbury, N.Y.: Health Education Literary Publishers, 1997), or consult your healthcare professional.

Pygeum

This herb is extracted from the bark of the African evergreen tree. Reputed for its ability to enhance the libido, pygeum is highly effective in treating symptoms of BPH. Pygeum works very well with saw palmetto, and the two herbs are often found formulated together. Users have reported a decrease in nighttime urination and interruption of normal urine flow.

Suggested Dose: 500 mg three times a day.

Saw Palmetto

Today in the U.S. saw palmetto is gaining more popularity as a viable option to Proscar™ in treating symptoms associated with BPH. Proscar™, as we've previously noted, works by inhibiting the activity of 5-alpha-reductase, responsible for the conversion of DHT (dihydrotestosterone) to testosterone. Numerous clinical trials (many conducted in Germany) have confirmed that saw palmetto is more effective in modulating the activity of 5-alpha-reductase. In fact, saw palmetto not only blocks the production of DHT, it actually inhibits DHT from adhering to cell-binding sites.

Why is this important? Well, this process—cell binding—could be compared to plugging an electrical cord into an appropriate outlet. However, imagine for the moment removing the cord and returning an hour later only to find that someone has put protective coverings over the outlet. Saw palmetto works like such a protective cover, which makes it more effective than Proscar™! By causing a roadblock, so to speak, at the cell-binding site, the door that allows DHT's entrance into the prostate cells is essentially closed. This unequivocally prevents prostate cells from absorbing testosterone and DHT.

Reports from Germany (specifically published reports by the Commission E) that detail saw palmetto's abilities have had an impact everywhere. The increased usage of saw palmetto in the U.S. has prompted officials to conduct the first ever International Saw Palmetto Symposium, in Naples, Florida in 1998, sponsored by The American Herbal Products Association of Bethesda, Maryland.

In addition to the above, saw palmetto plays a key role in controlling oxidative stress reactions within the prostate gland. Minimizing or neutralizing the trauma associated with oxidative stress (free-radical proliferation) is associated with proper function.

Suggested Dose: 300 to 500 mg, three times a day. Users of saw palmetto usually experience a diminished urinary urge and diminished nighttime urination within four to six weeks. Make sure your supplement is standardized to contain eighty-five to ninety-five percent fatty acids and sterols.

HORMONES

Hormones are internally secreted compounds formed in endocrine organs such as the liver and adrenal glands. Carried by body fluid to specific organs like the prostate gland, they play an essential role in a gland's proper functioning

DHEA

Over the last five years there has been an increased interest in Dehydroepiandrosterone—DHEA for short. Called the youth hormone, DHEA is the most abundant hormone in the human body. DHEA acts as an antioxidant and is responsible for helping the body adapt to stress, make sex hormones, modulate immune function, inhibit harmful (LDL) cholesterol buildup, and discourage the development of cancer.

Levels of DHEA dramatically decline with age. Low levels have been implicated in the development of many of today's long-term degenerative diseases. According to C. Norman Shealy, M.D., founder and director of the Shealy Institute for Comprehensive Healthcare in Springfield, Missouri and author of *DHEA: The Youth and Health Hormone,* every type of cancer that has been studied has some correlation to low levels of DHEA.

Dr. Shealy states that if a male has a baseline blood level of DHEA below 750 ng/dl anytime after age thirty or forty, by far the most important thing he can do is to restore DHEA levels to optimal ranges. (p. 41) For men, acceptable ranges are 750 ng/dl (nanograms per deciliter of blood).

DHEA can be purchased over the counter, usually in dose ranges of 25–50 mg. Do not exceed these ranges as a daily supplement, since DHEA will convert into testosterone.

7-Keto DHEA
7-Keto DHEA is a relatively new supplement. It is a derivative of the hormone DHEA just discussed. However, 7-Keto DHEA will not convert to testosterone, while giving you all of the benefits of DHEA. 7-Keto DHEA can boost your libido, offer protection as a free-radical scavenger and enhance overall immune function.

In a related matter, *Natural Pharmacy News* (April 1999, pp. 1–2) reported that researchers at the University of Wisconsin discovered that 7-Keto DHEA can increase production of interleukin-2 (IL-2) by 103 percent, as compared to 88 percent using DHEA. Interleukin-2 is produced by those cells in the bone marrow that scientists call CD-4. You could call CD-4 cells the ground-troop forces sent in to immobilize hostile immune system invaders. T-suppressor cells, known as CD-8, then round up any viruses, parasites or cancerous cells missed in the initial attack by the immune system.

Interleukin-2 production, enhanced by 7-Keto DHEA, acts as a backup alarm system that signals the immune system that its initial forces have been penetrated by the enemy, thus requiring reinforcements. For the individual concerned about maintaining proper prostate function, or slowing down the negative spiral of deteriorating prostate health, 7-Keto DHEA may offer significant help.

Suggested Dose: 25 mg, three times a day.

NATURAL ACCESSORY SUPPLEMENTS

Beta-1, 3 D-Glucan

This new supplement is being heralded as one of the most powerful macrophage activators occurring in nature. Made from a simple sugar from the cell wall of an ordinary yeast known as *saccharomyces cerevisiae,* Beta-1,3 D-Glucan is now available in supplement form. Macrophages are a form of white blood cells (originally made in the bone marrow) that act as internal scavengers. They scour the internal terrain, literally engulfing and eating up cancer cells and other harmful agents that could cause the immune system to malfunction. Beta-1,3 D-Glucan could be compared to a city sanitation and maintenance department. The target of Beta-1,3 D-Glucan, however, would be to clean up and destroy anything that would harm healthy tissue and cells.

To learn more about the optimum dose necessary to be most effective, Dr. Kenneth Hunter, Jr., vice-president for research at the University of Nevada School of Medicine in Reno, recently announced the award of a $100,000 grant to study Beta-Glucan further. The research project is entitled, "Investigation of the Mode of Action of Beta-Glucan Immuno-potentiator."

Note: Beta-1,3 D-Glucan can be purchased in vitamin and health stores under the name Macro Force. You can call 1-888-246-6839 for more information and the nearest retail location.

Suggested Dose: 7.5 mg, five times daily.

Cranberry

Supplementing the diet with cranberry in tablet, capsule or extract (liquid) form will help protect the urinary tract from infection. It is important to note that "extract form" does not refer to supermarket cranberry drinks or cranberry "cocktails." These products usually contain large amounts of sugar, and may actually encourage unwanted bacterial growth. Extract here refers to an herbal remedy that has been refined and occurs in its natural state.

By creating an acidic environment, cranberry prevents E-coli, the primary bacteria responsible for urinary tract infections, from adhering to walls of the urinary tract. Bacteria like E-coli adapt well in an alkaline or non-acidic environment.

Suggested Dose: Follow manufacturer's suggested dose range.

Modified Citrus Pectin

The inclusion of this supplement in your diet is one of the best things you could do for your prostate, both as a preventive and a treatment measure. Modified citrus pectin is a compound found in citrus fruits. Citrus pectin is found in fruit as long, imposing chains of sugar (carbohydrate) molecules. Modified citrus pectin has these same chains, but in much shorter lengths. Based on the pioneering work of Dr. Kenneth Pienta, Dr. David Platt and Dr. Avraham Raz of the Cancer Metastasis Program and the Michigan Cancer Foundation in Detroit, researchers now know that modified citrus pectin can inhibit the spreading of prostate cancer cells to other cites in the body. Dr. Pienta has stated that "To the best of our knowledge, this is the first report of an oral method to prevent spontaneous prostate cancer metastasis." (1996, p.16)

Modified citrus pectin in animal studies prohibited a group of proteins called lectins from attaching themselves to the walls of cancer cells. This is significant since lectins are the messenger cells that other cells use to communicate with one another. A lectin called galactin is found in abundance in prostate and other cancerous cells. Modified citrus pectin is used to destroy the message transmitted by prostate cancer cells, which is "Multipy."

Based on current knowledge, there is no safety issue of intake with this harmless fruit product. Modified citrus pectin can be purchased over the counter at local vitamin and health stores.

Suggested Dose: As a daily protective supplement, 1 to 5 grams daily. For individuals diagnosed with prostate cancer, 5 to 10 grams daily.

Note: Due to the high incidence of prostate-related disorders among African-American males, I highly recommend that this supplement be used by men of African descent as early as age twenty-five.

Sex

Although sex is not an actual supplement, sex in moderation is good for the prostate gland. This is not to imply that sexual intercourse can alleviate prostate disturbances; however, during ejaculation, unwanted stagnation and sedimentation of prostatic fluid is prevented, thus reducing oxidative stress within the prostate gland. This is good!

Researchers like Richard Milsten, M.D., former chief of Urology at Underwood-Memorial Hospital and Medical Director of the Center for Sexual Health in Woodbury, New Jersey, state that "males who experience sexual activity earlier in life and more frequently are more likely to retain their potency in later years." (p. 182) In a related note, Joseph Poticha, M.D., a former clinical professor of Obstetrics-Gynecology and a marriage and sex counselor at the Center for Marital and Sexual Studies at Northwestern University, maintains that masturbating is another way to keep your tissues vital.

Shark Cartilage

This substance was made known to the general public through a book by William Lane, Ph.D., called *Sharks Don't Get Cancer.* Shark cartilage is touted for its antiangiogenesis capabilities. (To refresh your memory, an antiangiogenic substance prevents cancer cells from forming the new blood vessels they need to survive.)

Suggested Dose: 500 to 800 mg, three to four times daily.

Water

While you may not consider water to be a supplement, I consider it to be an accessory nutrient.

Many males do not consume enough clean, fresh water. Water helps flush the kidneys of toxins, thus reducing the work of the liver. You should drink eight to ten glasses of clean, fresh water daily. This will increase urination and preventing excess debris and toxins from finding their way to the prostate gland. Additionally, dehydration stresses the prostate, possibly leading to inflammation.

VITAMINS AND MINERALS

Like enzymes, vitamins and minerals are part of the body's labor force. Known as "catalysts," they help speed up reactions which, without their help, occur too slowly to support life processes such as proper prostate function.

Vitamin C

Vitamin C is one of the most well-known and widely-used supplements in the U.S. Made famous by the late Dr. Linus Pauling, the Nobel Prize-winning chemist, vitamin C has, in recent years, received much attention due to its antioxidant capabilities. There also has been renewed interest in vitamin C's anti-cancer and immune system abilities in the treatment and prevention of prostate disorders. According to Dr. Pauling, cancer patients generally exhibit a decreased effectiveness of their natural immune-protective mechanisms. His recommendation:

> The simplest and safest way to enhance immunocompetence in these patients and to ensure that their molecular and cell-mediated defense systems are working at maximum efficiency is to increase their intake of vitamin C. (1979, p. 111)

As a preventive as well as a restorative measure I strongly recommend the "vitamin C flush." This cleansing procedure should be done once a month. It is an invaluable, safe and inexpensive way to build resistance, detoxify the system and destroy harmful bacteria. This is vital to anyone concerned with good prostate health, since, as previously discussed, the prostate gland seems to be a gathering site for harmful bacterial.

To do the vitamin C flush:

1. Mix 1000 mg of powdered vitamin C in a cup of water.

2. Drink the above dosage every half-hour until you reach a point of experiencing mild diarrhea. **Note:** This is your marker for the range that is tolerable by your system.

3. Omit one of your dosages right up to the point of your diarrhea, and take this dose every four hours for one or two days. For instance, if you took six, 1000 mg doses and then experienced diarrhea, that means you took 6000 mg. Omit one—which means your dose is 5000 mg—and take this amount every four hours for a day or two.

Repeat once a month. As a daily supplement, take 1000 to 3000 mgs. For optimal health, or in cases of weakened immune function, take 3000 to 5000 mgs daily.

Vitamin E

Vitamin E, like vitamin C, is one of the most widely-used vitamins, having withstood ridicule as a preventive nutrient against heart disease. It has finally gained recognition as a preventive factor in the development of disturbances of circulation, oxidative stress, and the buildup of free radicals—all of which contribute to heart disease.

A recent study jointly done by the U.S. National Cancer Institute and the University of Helsinki, Finland, showed that 50 mgs a day of vitamin E, supplemented orally, reduced a man's risk of developing prostate cancer by thirty-three percent. The study looked at the advancement of prostate cancer of 29,000 male smokers, aged fifty to sixty-nine. Mortality among the subjects also decreased by forty-one percent. The men in this study were tracked for eight years. (Cited briefly by Perlmutter, 1998. Further details can be found in *The Lancet,* March 28, 1998.)

In a related study, Philip Taylor, M.D., of the National Cancer Institute, reported that in a trial consisting of 14,564 men, those who took vitamin E experienced thirty-two percent fewer prostate cancer deaths. Researchers concluded that vitamin E may help prevent existing prostate cancer tumors from developing into a more aggressive form. (*Journal of the National Cancer Institute,* March 18, 1998)

Selenium

This trace mineral has only recently (since 1990) been recognized as essential to health. Selenium works synergistically with vitamin E to form one of the body's most potent anti-cancer and anti-aging enzymes. This enzyme, glutathione peroxidase, could be compared to an elite force of commandos whose job is to eradicate uncontrolled free radicals. Free radicals have been implicated as causative factors of prostate cancer and other age-related degenerative diseases. Daily dosages of 200 micrograms (mcgs) have produced dramatic reductions in the development of prostate cancers. In fact, studies have shown that men who supplement their diet with 200 mcg of selenium daily have two-thirds less chance of developing prostate cancer. (*Journal of the American Medical Association*, Dec. 25, 1996)

Similar results were also found by researchers at the University of Arizona, who detailed the results of a study of 974 men who took 200 mcgs of selenium for 4.5 years. These scientists found a sixty-three percent reduction in the risk of developing prostate cancer. (Clark, 1998)

Researchers at the University of Nebraska Medical Center found that even small amounts of selenium will activate natural killer cells. This finding should be viewed as monumental, since NK cells are somewhat dormant as cancer progresses.

It is important to note that selenium's anti-cancer attributes are severely hampered without generous amounts of vitamin E present in the bloodstream and tissues.

Suggested Dose: 200 mcg daily.

Zinc

Used by millions in lozenge form to fight the common cold, zinc's efficacy as a valuable option in the prevention and treatment of prostate disturbances has also been well documented.

Besides enhancing immune function, zinc is involved in the inhibition of DHT conversion to testosterone. Furthermore, zinc plays a critical role as an antioxidant responsible for decreasing the formation of free radicals in the body. Present in semen, zinc is the most abundant mineral found in the prostate. There is evidence that zinc has the ability to reduce the size of the prostate, thus reducing the symptoms associated with BPH. (Leake et al., 1984)

Individuals suffering from prostate disorders are encouraged to consume generous amounts of *seronoa serrulata,* commonly known as pumpkin seeds, due to their high zinc content.

Suggested Dose: 50 to 100 mg daily.

Note: Due to zinc's poor absorption rate, I recommend that you take it in lozenge form. Also, according to urologist Dr. James Balch, zinc needs pyridoxine (vitamin B-6) present to be properly metabolized and converted to a form that can be easily absorbed by the prostate gland.

WHOLE FOOD FACTORS
Chlorella

Chlorella is known and used in alternative medical circles as a cell rejuvenator and oxygenator. Part of the family of whole foods known as "green gold" because of their rich chlorophyll content, chlorella also has powerful anti-cancer capabilities. Benjamin Lau, M.D., Ph.D., of the Department of Microbiology, School of Medicine at Loma Linda University, California, maintains that chlorella plays a key role in initiating a process known as the "oxidative burst."

The oxidative burst could be compared to the force and impact that occurs at the line of scrimmage in a football game when a back tries to turn the corner, only to be met head on by two or three charging linebackers. According to Dr. Lau, at the completion of this oxidative burst by the macrophage, the decomposition of the foreign invader is followed by the emission of light. This light can be tracked and measured scientifically by a measurement known as chemiluminescence (CL). Forget the jargon here, but it is important to remember that scientists like Dr. Lau have discovered that an increase in CL activity via external stimulation (as with chlorella) correlates with an increased assault on pathogenic microorganisms and tumor cells by the immune system.

Due to the slow development of BPH and its related disorders, chlorella, with its capacity to stimulate macrophage activity, is a valuable addition to your supplement routine.

Suggested Dose: 600 to 1200 mg daily.

Essential Fatty Acids

With most fat-laden diets the chances of developing heart disease, arthritis, breast and prostate cancer, as well as other chronic degenerative diseases, increases. On the other hand, fat is a healthy staple of the Japanese diet, as well as that of Greenland and Alaskan Eskimos. These populations consume docosahexaenoic (DHA) and eicosapentaeonic acid, known as EPA—the good fats or unsaturated fats. DHA and EPA are found in fish oils, soy oil, flax oil, black currant oil and safflower oil. These essential fatty acids can reduce the severity of symptoms or complications associated with BPH.

There is evidence that flaxseed oil is altered in the human gastrointestinal tract into an anti-cancer compound (Adlercreutz et al., 1986). Supplementation or consumption of DHA and EPA (fish oils) has resulted in increased lymphocyte recognition and consequent destruction of cancer cells. (Cooper, 1998, p. 24) This effect, according to researchers Ewan Cameron and Linus Pauling (1979) is due to the role that essential fatty acids and vitamin C play in producing prostaglandin PGE1. Prostaglandins are hormone-like substances that are intimately involved with the function of T-lymphocytes—the immune defenders that specifically target the destruction of cancer cells.

Suggested Dose: Follow the manufacturer's guidelines when using any of the supplemental forms of essential fatty acids.

Lycopene

Lycopene is the photonutrient that gives tomatoes their bright red color. Results of a recent study at Harvard University Medical School have confirmed lycopene's protective effect against prostate cancer. This tomato-based carotenoid (not to be confused with Beta-carotene) may reduce a man's risk of developing prostate cancer by thirty-five percent.

In the above study (which appeared in the *Journal of the National Cancer Institute,* Dec. 6, 1995), researchers looked at the effects of lycopene on 47,894 men aged forty to seventy-five. These men were free of prostate cancer at the start of the study. Between 1986 and 1992, twelve cases of prostate cancer were noted in the study group. The incidence of prostate cancer was then correlated to the overall intake of lycopene-based products.

The study tracked the dietary preferences of the men in the group for six years, assessing the intake of over 131 foods and beverages. The researchers found that tomato sauce, tomatoes, pizza and strawberries reduced prostate cancer risk by thirty-five percent. This occurrence was seen in those men who consumed ten or more servings of the first three foods a week.

At the Annual Meeting of the American Association for Cancer Research (April 1999, Philadelphia, Pennsylvania), Omer Kucuk, M.D., an oncologist from the Barbara Ann Karmanos Cancer Institute in Detroit, Michigan, presented evidence that lycopene may not only help prevent the development of prostate cancer, but actually be beneficial in treating men diagnosed with the disease. Dr. Kucuk and his associates found that after three weeks of supplementation with 15 mgs of lycopene twice daily, PSA levels dropped dramatically. These researchers also reported that lycopene prevented the spread of prostate cancer cells. ("Lycopene Study Shows Promise Against Cancer." *Vitamin Retailer.* East Brunswick, New Jersey: June 1999, vol. 6, no. 6)

Medicinal Mushrooms

Mushrooms have long been used in traditional Japanese and Chinese medicine as natural immune system activators and anti-cancer agents. Medicinal mushrooms (such as the shiitake and maitake) contain generous amounts of Beta-glucan, a compound we reviewed earlier. Shiitake mushrooms, used extensively in China, can stimulate T-cell activity. These cells help defend against foreign invaders as well as normalize liver function, which is essential to internal detoxification.

Maitake mushrooms from Japan have shown the ability to stop the process of angiogenesis, thus preventing cancer from spreading from one internal body site to another. As we have learned, cancer needs new blood vessels to survive.

THE AUTHOR'S RECOMMENDATIONS

As you can see, there is ongoing research concerning the efficacy of natural supplements as both a preventive and treatment tool for BPH and cancer of the prostate. When setting up a supplement plan it is important that you discuss your intentions with your physician and stay focused on your individual goals so you will not become overwhelmed with the plethora of supplements on the market today. In your quest to find the right combination or group of supplements, remember the words "trial and error." In many cases it may take four to six weeks to see any appreciable results from supplements. Natural supplements work by augmenting normal metabolic cycles, not by overriding them. In this way balance is restored instead of causing some other metabolic malfunction to occur.

As a basic regimen to support proper prostate function I would recommend that the following combination of supplements be taken daily:

1. A high potency or mega-multivitamin and mineral formula
2. Saw palmetto and pygeum
3. A multi-enzyme supplement
4. Modified citrus pectin
5. Lycopene
6. Additional vitamin C, E, and selenium
7. Lipoic acid

Note: The above are merely recommendations. They are not written in stone, meaning that you have the option to build a plan based on your individual needs. For those who have been diagnosed with prostate cancer, your needs may vary greatly in reference to the dose ranges presented here. This should be thoroughly discussed with your healthcare professional, as each case must be evaluated on an individual basis.

CONCLUSION

It is important to remember that supplements have a long history of use, in some cases over 5,000 years. Unlike drugs, these natural compounds can be taken as single entities or part of a multi-formulation. The beauty of natural supplementation is the synergistic effect of combining supplements versus using a single supplement alone. For example, the combination of saw palmetto and pygeum produces a stronger effect than either alone, as does the combination of vitamin E and the mineral selenium, and that of zinc and vitamin B-6.

Do not be swayed by erroneous reports about the dangers of supplements. There is a worldwide movement toward the use of safer alternatives to dangerous prescription drugs to treat disorders of the prostate and other long-term degenerative diseases. The fact is that every year ten million Americans have some sort of negative reaction to prescription and over-the-counter drugs. It is becoming apparent that we have been frantically looking for health in the wrong place. The use of "natural born medicaments" is becoming part of our social as well as our moral fabric.

In the next chapter, "Proper Nutrition As Preventive Medicine," we will take a look at how individual food preferences can contribute to the strength or the deterioration of the prostate gland.

CHAPTER SEVEN

PROPER NUTRITION
AS PREVENTIVE MEDICINE

Nutrients are what the human body has to work with in building
and maintaining healthy cells, tissues, glands, and organs. All
the other modalities, be it drugs, surgery, manipulations,
acupuncture, hydro-electro-magneto-therapy—you name it!—
can be useful and have their place in the arsenal of treatments,
but they fail in most cases unless the corrective and supportive
nutritional therapy is given priority.

—*Paavo Airola, Ph.D., N.D.*

While Jeffrey Bland, Ph.D., a nationally known professor of Nutritional Biochemistry and former director of the Linus Pauling
Institute of Health states that, "it is not fair to suggest that all
major diseases are caused by suboptimal nutrition,"(p.1), there
is mounting evidence that many of today's long-term degenerative diseases are a direct result of poor nutritional habits. This
theory had been extensively researched by Emanuel Cheraskin,
M.D. Dr. Cheraskin and associates, in their epic *Diet and Disease*
(1966 and 1987), presented scientific evidence that conclusively
showed that there was a direct link between improper dietary
habits and the onset of disease. The evidence of this link, although venomously disputed by his medical colleagues, has
always been there, according to Dr. Cheraskin. "Although

101

largely ignored, the evidence was right in the publications of the *American Medical Association*, the *American Dental Association*, the *American Journal of Clinical Nutrition*, and the *New England Journal of Medicine*, as well as in numerous other standard texts and conventional periodicals, meaning medical publications." The insidious paradox is that although not enough has changed in reference to recognizing the evidence, more of it has accumulated supporting the connection between improper diet and disease.

Dr. Airola's opening quote implies that no healing can take place until the problem of improper nutrition is fully addressed. This same sentiment is expressed by Dr. Uno Erasmus known as the "fat doctor." Dr. Erasmus, a well-known authority on the clinical application of fats and oils in human nutrition, and author of *Fats that Heal, Fats that Kill*, explains that the entire human body (including your prostate gland) is made from food, air and water. (1988, p.1)

Dr. James Balch notes that the rising incidence of prostate cancer, especially those men diagnosed in their forties and fifties, is a direct result of improper dietary considerations and increased exposure to environmental toxins. Robyn Landis, the author of *Herbal Defense*, insists that the maintenance of health was meant to be a simple task:

> At the most basic level, health maintenance is relatively simple: Provide the body with what it needs, don't give it much of what it doesn't need, and the body will run itself. (p. 325)

However, in today's society, this simple task is becoming increasingly difficult. Sherry Rogers, M.D., who specializes in environmental medicine, claims that the human body today is subjected to an array of chemicals and pesticides that were not part of our environmental landscape in years past.

So, it would seem that those old adages, "An apple a day keeps the doctor away," and "Let thy food be thy medicine," are backed by scientific evidence. Brian L. Morgan, M.D., a faculty member at the Institute of Human Nutrition at Columbia University College of Physicians and Surgeons, states that "it has become increasingly clear that dietary changes—that is, the practice of preventive nutrition—can contribute to improved health and the prevention of disease." (1987, p.viii)

PROPER NUTRITION

This simple concept of giving the body more of what it needs is vital to the maintenance of good prostate health. By doing this all of your internal systems will function much more efficiently. Overloading the body with excessive amounts of the wrong kinds of fuel (food) will only interfere with normal metabolic cycles.

We are made up of a diverse system of cells that grow, multiply, and eventually die. However, dead cells can be replaced by new energy-filled cells. If what you give your system is good wholesome food in its proper ratio, this process is enhanced. Your prostate gland as well as your other internal systems can be refurbished much more efficiently. Furthermore, in this beautifully orchestrated process, as the body is rebuilding, the removal of waste and harmful by-products of metabolism is accelerated. To do this the body needs energy. The driving force behind this process is our diet.

Imagine for a moment how well your car runs after it has been tuned up. If you regularly use high-test gasoline, remember what happened to that powerful thrust when you switched to a low-grade formula. In an extreme example, remember what happened when you put oil in your gas tank instead of the engine.

If you can begin to view your prostate gland in the same way as you might view your car, you can begin to understand why proper nutrition is your first line of defense. Understand from this standpoint, it becomes apparent why alternative healthcare professionals believe that the individual controls his potential to remain free of prostate trouble.

PREVENTIVE NUTRITION

Can proper nutrition prevent, correct or slow-down the associated complications of benign prostate hyperplasia or prostate cancer? From all indications, this may be a possibility. Past and present data have confirmed (although still disputed, albeit with less voracity) that one's dietary preferences can contribute greatly to the development of prostate dysfunction. "Germs" today are not our principle enemy. Our chief medical adversary is the disturbance of the inner balance of the constituents of our tissues, which are built from and maintained by the food and water we drink, and the chemicals in the air that we breathe.

While nutritional factors alone shouldn't be considered the answer, they should be viewed as your first line of defense against prostate disturbances. When approached from this context you are practicing preventive nutrition, which could be defined as a nutritional protocol designed to change, maintain, or encourage an internal environment that is able to defend itself.

From our discussion thus far it becomes apparent that the raw materials the body uses to rebuild and sustain itself come from the food we eat. This fact that proper nutrition is the body's first line of defense still seems to elude many medical professionals, and is not totally understood by the general population. It is ironic that what we in the U.S. call preventive nutrition is standard in many countries of world. For example, in Japan, consumption of soy rich foods, reduced animal protein (from red meats) and less saturated fats is common practice. Men who migrate to the United States from Japan and African countries and adopt the "normal" American diet, risk a significant rise in their chances of developing prostate cancer. In fact, autopsies done worldwide reveal that wherever dietary habits are closely related to that of Americans (characterized by high animal fat consumption), close to twenty-five percent of all men develop prostate cancer. (Robbins, p. 270)

A SIMPLE TASK

As previously stated, the maintenance of health was meant to be a simple task—give the body a lot of what it needs and little of what it doesn't. Although we know this statement is true, here in the United States we tend to give the body a lot of what it doesn't need. For example, the bulk of our diet consists of red meat, milk, eggs, cheeses, and saturated fats. All of these foods in excess promote the development of all types of cancer, including prostate cancer. This is why many researchers insist that macrobiotic and vegetarian-type diets are excellent as preventive measures. For example, studies conducted with the Seventh-Day Adventists in the United States show that they suffer far less cancer than the general population. About one half of all Seventh-Day Adventists are vegetarians.

BECOME YOUR OWN NUTRITIONIST

It is now known that forty percent of all men's cancers, including prostate cancer, are caused by nutritional factors alone. (Simone, p. 113) If this is the case, why don't medical doctors insist that their patient's adhere to this simple preventive measure. Well, as previously stated by Julian Whitaker, M.D., your doctor's job is to treat illness, not prevent it.

This premise was clarified in a 1983–84 survey conducted by the Association of American Medical Colleges Curriculum (AAMC) Directory. Over sixty percent of the medical students indicated that their nutrition education was inadequate. A large portion of the students (10,000) also reported (1981–1984) that the time spent on learning methods to prevent disease was insufficient. A big part of the problem is within the corridors of the majority of U.S. medical schools. Although the National Academy of Sciences suggests that medical students receive at least twenty-five hours of nutrition education, fewer than forty percent of all the medical schools in the U.S. that offer some nutritional education offer this required number of hours. The most insidious fact here, however, is that more than seventy-five percent of U.S. medical schools do not even offer courses in nutrition.

If your doctor is unable or unwilling to consider the possibility of improving your health by nutritional means you must become your own nutritionist.

As a society we have become enormously dependent on medical professionals in our quest to live disease free. Fortunately based on results from current data, this trend is rapidly changing. Stuart Berger, M.D., a graduate of Harvard University and author of *How to Be Your Own Nutritionist,* maintains that the perfect person to hire as your nutritionist is yourself. Dr. Berger claims that you know your nutritional habits better than anyone. I agree with his assessment because if you make the personal commitment to change your dietary habits, you actively take part in total control of your health—which is the way it should be.

Although the thought of becoming your own nutritionist may sound like an imposing task, especially since you have no formal nutritional training, nothing could be farther from the truth. You probably have the same if not more nutritional training than your personal physician. By remembering to take in a lot of what you need—like fruits, vegetables, nuts, seeds, fiber—and little of what the body doesn't need—red meats, milk, eggs, butter, and excessive protein—you can successfully chart your own nutritional course. Over consumption of the latter, known as "dead foods," will only burden normal metabolic activities. For example, red meats contain arachidonic acid, found also in dairy products and eggs, that causes cascades of free radicals to form. Arachidonic acid can also cause overstimulation of testosterone, which stimulates prostate cancer proliferation. Moreover, when red meat is consumed there is an increased production of white blood cells—a sign that the body is under attack.

Play the color game! Eat lots of green leafy vegetables and brightly colored fruits. Slowly exchange these for all those non-desirables. Personally, I do not advocate that you totally eliminate any food. Rather, I strongly recommend that you change your dietary patterns to coincide with the percentages below:

For Health Maintenance:

- ◆ 50% cooked fruits and vegetables
- ◆ 35% raw fruits and vegetables
- ◆ 15% grains, nuts, seeds, meat, dairy, or poultry.

This same sentiment is expressed by Robert Haas, Ph.D., a world-renowned nutritionist and author of *Permanent Remissions.* Dr. Haas says that you don't have to completely eliminate any food from your new way of eating, but you should drastically reduce your intake of the following foods in order to achieve optimal prostate health and a long-term or permanent remission from prostate cancer if you have it. (1997, p. 142) Haas recommends avoiding the following foods:

- ◆ red meat
- ◆ cheese
- ◆ vegetable oils (except olive oil, canola oil, omega-3 fish oils)
- ◆ ice cream
- ◆ whole milk
- ◆ mayonnaise
- ◆ butter
- ◆ egg yolks

NEW WAYS, NEW THINKING: THE ELEMENTS OF CHANGE

Claude Bernard, the famous nineteenth century researcher, in his quest to find the cause-and-effect relationship between food and its biological transmutation to sugar, found himself burdened with a theoretical dilemma. He had, through his own research, proved his hypothesis and theory wrong concerning the body's usage and storage of sugar and the onset of diabetes mellitus. The occurrence prompted him to make the following statement (Keravan, 1972):

> When one is confronted with a fact which is in opposition with a prevalent theory, one must accept this fact and abandon the theory, even though the latter, supported by great men and women, may be generally subscribed to.

The "new thinking" today focuses on a group of natural substances researchers have found in fruits and vegetables. Called photochemical, phytonutrients or nutraceuticals, these compounds are being investigated mainly due to their ability to disrupt the biochemical mechanism that allows prostate and other cancers to develop. Scientists are calling this phenomenon the "color wars."

It appears that those same bright colors or photochemicals that protect plants, fruits and vegetables from insects and the ravenges of sunlight, have the ability to prevent disease in humans, especially cancer. With the number of clinical trials being conducted, and the positive results, there is new thinking concerning nutrition and its medical application, so much so that the prestigious U.S. National Cancer Institute recently established a $20.5 million dollar program to study phytochemicals.

THE PROOF'S IN THE PUDDING

Just what are investigators finding in the simple soybean, grape seeds, fruits, dried beans, tomatoes, broccoli, sweet potatoes, and colorful cruciferous vegetables. The following table will give you a concise look at which phytonutrients are found in which foods, their scientific names and how they work in the body.

ASSESSING YOUR OWN NUTRITIONAL STATUS

With any new project it is always best to formulate an action plan. By doing this you can get an overall picture of where you are presently, and where you would like to be. Also, as the word "action" implies, the plan (via an organized sequence of events) can move you to a more desirable plateau. To get started I suggest you do the following:

1. Conduct a Diet Survey

By conducting a diet survey of your individual dietary habits, you are better equipped to make gradual changes.

2. Have Biochemical Testing Done

Knowing where you stand in reference to your individual biochemistry is vital to maintaining good prostate function. What is

NATURAL FOOD PROTECTORS

Protector	Food	Protective Action
Carotene	Carrots, sweet potatoes, yams, pumpkins, squash kale, broccoli, cantaloupe	Neutralizes free radicals and singlet oxygen radicals; enhances immune systems; reverses pre-cancer conditions; high intake associated with low cancer rates
Indole	Cabbage family: cabbage, broccoli, cauliflower, mustard greens, etc.	Destroys estrogen, known to initiate new cancers, mustard, greens, etc. especially breast cancer
Isoflavones	Legumes: beans, peas, peanuts	Inhibits estrogen action; inhibits prostaglandin, hormones that cause cancer spread
Lignans	Flaxseed, walnuts, fatty fish	Inhibits estrogen action; inhibits prostaglandin, hormones that cause cancer spread
Polyacetylene	Parsley	Inhibits prostaglandin; destroys benzopyrene, a potent carcinogen
Protease Inhibitors	Soybeans	Destroys enzymes that can cause cancer to spread.
Quinones	Rosemary	Inhibits carcinogens or co-carcinogens
Sterols	Cucumbers	Decreases cholesterol
Sulfur	Garlic	Inhibits carcinogens, inhibits cancer spread, decreases cholesterol
Terpenes	Citrus fruit	Increases enzymes to break down carcinogens; decreases cholesterol
Triterpenoids	Licorice	Inhibits estrogens, prostaglandins; slows down rapidly dividing cells, like cancer cells

Source: Charles B. Simone, M.D., *Cancer and Nutrition.* Garden Park City, N.Y: Avery Publishing Group, Inc. (800–548–5757), 1992, p. 127. Used by permission.

your current cholesterol blood status? What is your triglyceride count, pH status and gamma-glutamyl transpeptidase (GGTP) status. An elevation in GGTP in the blood may be a signal that you are not able to properly metabolize alcohol. This is bad news for your prostate gland.

3. Test for Food Allergies

While proper nutrition is important, sensitivity to certain foods can tax the system. This causes the immune system to work overtime, and can cause free radical proliferation. These undesirables have a way of taking up residence within the prostate gland.

4. Get Help

I would strongly suggest you find a certified nutritionist who specializes in environmental medicine. There are about 25,000 registered pesticide products worldwide. Agricultural use of pesticides has increased 170 percent over the last eighteen years, which has affected the nutrient quality of our food supply.

In your efforts to find the right balance of nutrients, finding a certified nutritionist or health professional who specializes in environmental medicine may be of great benefit. Please refer to Chapter Nine, for assistance in finding the right practitioner for you.

5. Study

To also assist you in your efforts, I highly recommend the following books:

Bieler, H.G., *Food Is Your Best Medicine,* New York: Random House, 1968.

Berger, S., *How To Be Your Own Nutritionist,* New York: William Morrow and Co., 1968.

Bricklin, M., and Claessens, S. *The Natural Healing Cookbook,* Emmaus, Penn.: Rodale Press, 1981.

Claessens, S., *The 20-Minute Natural Foods Cookbook,* Emmaus, Penn., Rodale Press, 1982.

Dixon, B.M., *Good Health For African Americans,* New York: Crown Publishers, 1994.

Haas, R., *Permanent Remissions,* New York: Simon and Schuster, Inc., 1997.

Hausman, P., *Foods That Fight Cancer,* New York: Rawson Associates, 1983.

Mindell, E., *Unsafe At Any Meal,* New York: Warner Books, 1987.

Nixon, D.W., *The Cancer Recovery Eating Plan,* New York: Random House, 1994.

Salaman, M., *Foods That Heal,* Menlo Park, Calif.: James Stafford Publishing, 1996.

THE DO EAT DIET

Over the years all of us have developed individual food preferences. The hardest thing to do for many of us is to break or change habits that have become a daily part of our lives. Food choices are such a personnel preference and many of us resent being told what not to eat. Nonetheless, proper nutrition is the most important variable in your quest to remain free of prostate disturbances.

I am going to list some "Do Eats" for you. But before I do that I would like you to start a Food Diary. In this diary, which could be done in a regular composition book or a loose-leaf binder, you keep a record of all the different foods you eat day by day, and the quantity.

Food Diary

Use one page for each day's recordings, and keep the diary for thirty days. Start by dividing the first page into sections according to the categories of food you eat, such as fruits (raw and cooked), vegetables (raw and cooked), cereals, grains, breads, desserts, meats, dairy, poultry, alcoholic beverages and other beverages. Put today's date on this first page. Note all that you eat today in the appropriate area. For instance, under vegetables you might record: *large green salad with tomatoes, onions, cucumbers.*

At the end of thirty days you will have accumulated a lot of valuable information about your diet. Take a broad overview and look for patterns. For instance, look for individual days or consecutive days where fiber intake was low or absent, or where vegetable and fruit consumption was nonexistent. Note the consumption of your "favorite dishes," which may be quite unhealthy.

Once you have established what, where and when this pattern is occurring, I would like you to start breaking this chain of negative eating habits by doing the following for a period of two weeks.

1. Start a new *Food Diary.* Use the same food categories, except eliminate alcohol. Replace with nonalcoholic beer, if necessary.

2. Take a trip to your local library and check out a few books that cover such subjects as low-fat cooking ideas; cancer and proper nutrition; high fiber foods; fresh vegetable juice and herb tea; vegetarian or macrobiotic diets; organic foods; soy foods; health tonics and natural foods.

3. Contact the American Diatetic Association and ask them to send you information concerning the Food Exchange Program they have developed. (In the U.S., phone: 800-ADA-DISC, ext. 363.)

4. At the end of a two-week period take a serious look at the information you are gathering on the foods you can and should be eating. Refer to my "Do Eat" list (which follows) to assist you in beginning one of your own.

5. Start exchaning the "bad guys"—high-fat, low fiber foods—for the "good guys."

6. Repeat this process again in three months, and then three months after that.

After completing the *Food Diary* process several times you will realize how easily we get into what I call a "food rut." Many times we fall into the familiar pattern of eating only those foods that we have been accustomed to from childhood.

By formulating your own "Do Eat" list you are actually charting your own nutritional preferences, much like I did and have done in my quest to remain cancer free. The beauty of the "Do Eat" list is that you will be contributing to removing a major obstacle to cure and health maintenance, namely, your own dietary choices.

Do Eat:

1. Two to three cups of fruit daily, preferably raw
2. A bowl of oat-bran cereal every morning
3. Three to four servings of fresh vegetables daily. Introduce new veggies into your routine
4. Fish, chicken, and turkey. It is okay to occasionally eat prime rib, steak, or beef
5. Herbal teas and Chinese green tea
6. Flaxseed, olive, canola, or peanut oils
7. Soy, rice, or goat's milk
8. Pinto beans, navy beans, green peas, kidney beans, black-eyed beans, lima beans, red beans
9. Fructose and blackstrap molasses sweeteners
10. Potassium chloride-type seasonings
11. Brazil nuts, walnuts, soybeans, pumpkin seeds, pecans
12. Sweet potatoes, tomatoes
13. Whole-grain pasta, brown rice, bran, wheat germ, rice
14. Soy grits, soy cheese, soy flour, soy pancake mix
15. Dressing made with olive or canola oil
16. Yogurt, sherbet
17. Fresh fruit juice

Note: Try to eat four to five mini-meals instead of two or three large meals. This is better for proper digestive and metabolic functions.

CONCLUSIONS

From our discussion here it should become apparent that *you* are the most important variable to managing and preventing prostate disturbances. The exciting part of this equation is the meager economic cost involved. You do not have to spend thousands of dollars on prescription medications. Many of the preventive agents that progressive researchers have discovered are found at your local grocery store. You now have a solid base of nutritional information to start charting your own preventive nutritional profile against BPH or prostate cancer.

You also have enough nutritional knowledge to make the right choices. It is, however, advisable to get feedback and guidance about your plan from a qualified health professional, especially if you have been diagnosed with prostate cancer. The key in whatever decision you make is consistency and adherence to the guidelines previously outlined. If you want to permanently reap the rewards of a lifetime of good prostate health, make no mistake about it, a solid nutritional program is the way to prevention. You only need to make the commitment!

PART FOUR

Managing Prostate Health

If I would have known that I was going to live this long, I would have taken better care of myself.

—*Mickey Mantle*

CHAPTER EIGHT

DESIGNING A PERSONAL MAINTENANCE PLAN

We are convinced that every disease, physical and mental is generated by a combination of circumstances which are both inside and outside the body. It logically follows that disease may be prevented or cured by correcting variables that exist both inside and outside the body: *we can go after the "germ," but we need also to correct the life condition which predisposed the individual to illness.*

—*E. Cheraskin, M.D.* and
W.M. Ringsdorf, D.M.D.

While the late, great, New York Yankee Hall of Famer, Mickey Mantle will always be remembered for his contribution on and off the field of baseball, his remark on the preceding page was inspiring to me. His words refocused my effort toward maintaining optimal health. They also tie in with the above quote from Cheraskin and Ringsdorf. "To correct the life condition which predisposed the individual to illness" has a powerful connotation. It squarely puts the responsibly for health maintenance on the shoulders of the individual.

Patrick Walsh asked a series of probing questions back in Chapter One. Those questions were:

- ◆ Why do some men live for nearly a century without suffering from an enlarged prostate, while others from middle age onward, need to be treated more than once?
- ◆ Why do some men die with prostate cancer, and other men die of it—while others never get the disease?

The answer to the last question is intimately intertwined with your current lifestyle, your hereditary background, and the power of your immune system. In the April 1992 issue of *Health Magazine,* an article titled "Cheating Fate" asked: "At death's door, some people mysteriously take a turn for the better. What does the body know that medicine can't explain?"

To take this phenomenon a step farther, notice when you review the Naturopathic Model of Health and Disease that follows, that somewhere between optimal health and collapse of the vital force certain stressors cause a negative spiral in which health is eventually compromised. (See Figure 8.1)

According to T. Michael Culp, N.D., adjunct faculty member at Bastyr University in Seattle, the persistent presence of stressors in the body produces inflammation at the microscopic level. If the body is well nourished, however, circulating and eliminating properly, the stressors are easily neutralized. (p.47) Poor lifestyle habits can accelerate the actions of these stressors, impeding proper circulation, thus leading to chronic degeneration and consequent dysfunction of inborn metabolic mechanisms. Stressors can be psychological stress, a tumor, poor enzyme function, clogged arteries, among other things.

How efficiently your body is able to neutralize these every day assaults will go a long way toward preserving prostate health. How well you are able to cope mentally also has a direct bearing on overall health. Robert Sorge, Ph.D.,N.D., director of the Abunda Life Health Hotel and Clinic in Asbury Park, N.J., states that positive attitudes are as much a nourishment to our bodies as vitamins and minerals. As you probably know, medical research has confirmed the existence of an elite force of brain chemicals called endorphins. Secreted and used by the

HEALTH AND DISEASE: A NATUROPATHIC MODEL

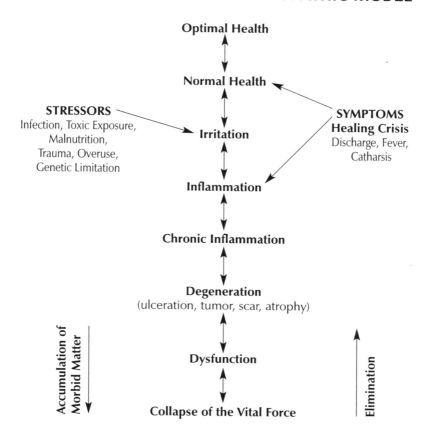

Figure 8.1 Source: "Naturopahtic Healing," Energy Times Magazine, Long Beach, Calif., July–Aug., 1996, p. 47. Used by permission. All rights reserved.

brain, endorphins help the body withstand pain and promote well-being. According to Dr. Sorge, we may soon learn that healthy people, those who experience high-level wellness, have an abundance of "natural opiates" like endorphins flowing in all parts of their body. (p.13)

The bottom line here is that optimism breeds health, and with it a strong immune response. What does all of this have to do with the prostate gland? Well, when you view prostate disorders from this perspective, you begin to realize that prostate disturbances are not simply confined to the prostate gland itself. You begin to realize that prostate problems are systemic disorders cause by varying factors. More importantly, once you understand all the ramifications that lead to dysfunction and the progression of the disorder, accepting that a comprehensive approach to managing and preventing prostate disturbances is needed becomes evident.

MORE FALSE TRUTHS

Once a man has been diagnosed with prostate cancer and/ or some sort of prostate disorder, is it then too late to start a health rebuilding or wellness program?

Nothing could be farther from the truth. You have the ability to correct past unhealthy lifestyles choices. In fact, your doctor, whether a conventional or an alternative physician, cannot protect you against the onset of prostate cancer, or any kind of cancer for that matter. According to Julian Whitaker, M.D.:

1. No drug can cut your chances of having arthritis or diabetes . . . **But you can!**

2. No hospital can protect you against heart attack or cancer . . . **But you can!**

3. No doctor can shield you from strokes or premature aging . . . **But you can!** (p. 4)

The present medical healthcare system in the U.S., although one of the best in the world, is a "for profit" entity. As such, its focus is on the treatment of disease, not on how to prevent it. Therefore, we must become our own advocates. Becoming your own advocate is not meant to imply that you try to diagnoses and design a treatment plan for what you believe to be some type of prostate disorder. In any plan of attack, it is imperative that you know the type of and the severity of the disorder you are dealing with. This can only be done in cooperation with your healthcare professional. As we have learned, one treatment or preventive plan does not fit all.

BUILDING AN INDESTRUCTIBLE PROSTATE GLAND

Gil Lederman, M.D., Director of Radiation Oncology at New York's Staten Island University Hospital states that many patients believe that once their radiation treatments are over the cancer cannot come back. This, according to Dr. Lederman, is not the case.

The point here is that one way or another you are going to have to develop some sort of wellness plan that is geared toward prevention. You will undoubtedly look at things differently, with the preservation of health likely becoming a major priority in your life, if medical intervention becomes necessary. My rise from the ashes, so to speak, after my bout with cancer certainly changed my focus from treatment to prevention measures designed for health preservation and nonrecurrence.

The problem, however, is that with the long-term degenerative nature of today's maladies such as heart disease, arthritis, and prostate disorders, preventive programs are not initiated until the disease has manifested. We must reject the false notion that "not hurting" and "healthy" are one and the same. If we begin to move away from that belief, it becomes apparent that the problem with combating many of today's degenerative diseases is not with the disease but ourselves.

This premise has also been echoed by Dr. Andrew Weil. His articles and books often reverberate with a strong message that health ought to flow from the way we live.

Wendy Fink, former consultant to the American Health Foundation and the U.S. Department of Health, Education and Welfare, and author of *Solving the Wellness Puzzle,* states that more than ninety-nine percent of us are born healthy. Yet over fifty percent of the deaths under the age of sixty-five can be directly attributed to the way we live. (p. 3)

The first step in any process geared toward prevention or recovery is a personal commitment toward change. In naturopathic medicine, refining the art of natural healing is crucial. What makes the naturopathic approach appealing is the goal of health maintenance, the commitment to prevention, and a dedication to teaching patients how to avoid sickness in the first place. Avoidance of disease, although not commonly practiced in many places, should be the cornerstone of all medicine.

This sentiment is strongly expressed by one of the most vocal advocates for the use of preventive and alternative measures to fight disease. The doctor once known as the "diet guru," Robert Atkins, when asked what his goals for the future were, responded by saying, "I want to see physicians as a group begin to practice medicine the way my Atkins Center physicians practice. We keep our patients out of hospitals, and get them well again. This is what I want to see before I retire." (p. 66)

As Nobel Prize winning scientist Rene Dubos said:

> Western medicine will become scientific only when physicians and their patients have learned to manage the forces of the body and the mind that operate in *vis medicatrix naturae.* (in Cummings and Ullman, p.10)

This ancient phrase, *vis medicatrix naturae,* means "the healing power of nature," and "refers directly to the human organism's dynamic and powerful capacity to protect and heal itself." (Cummings and Ullman, p. 10)

DR. REDMON'S 25 POINT PROSTATE WELLNESS PLAN

While the choice of treatment and the time length to employ it depend on a host of factors, there are, based on current scientist evidence, a plethora of preventive measures you can implement to prevent the onset, development or recurrence of prostate disturbances. While there is much controversy surrounding the efficacy of such programs, I strongly suggest that you do not become entangled in this controversy, as the residual benefits outweigh the inconsistencies of approval by many well-established organizations.

For example, it has only been recently acknowledged by the prestigious National Cancer Institute that diet conclusively plays a role in the prevention of cancer. Yet, for decades researchers have known that diet, as well as other factors, from environmental stress to the use of antihistamines, has contributed to the development of prostate dysfunction. Based on current scientific knowledge, I strongly recommend the inclusions of the 25 Point Plan that follows as a preventive measure in your quest to remain prostate-trouble free.

1. Eat more fiber.

2. Consume two to four servings of fresh fruit and three to five servings of a variety of fresh vegetables daily.

3. Reduce or eliminate red meat and fatty fried foods from your diet.

4. Develop a healthy sex relationship with your spouse or partner. The old adage, "Use it or lose it," should be taken literally when it comes to maintaining good pro-state health.

5. Reduce your exposure to pesticides and environmental pollutants.

6. Reduce your consumption of alcohol, especially beer. Beer increase the production of the hormone prolactin, and prolactin increases the uptake of testosterone by the prostate gland. This process greatly exacerbates BPH.

7. Stop smoking, and do not smoke and drink alcohol at the same time.

8. Drink at least eight glasses of clean, fresh water a day.

9. Begin using saw palmetto or other natural extracts known to support prostate health and function.

10. Become an activist—that is, keep moving, and incorporate exercise into your life. Walking is very good for maintaining prostate health.

11. Chart your personal health history and that of your immediate and first-line family members.

12. Lose some weight.

13. Ask questions, read, listen, and learn. Become familiar with the associated risk factors of prostate disease and take appropriate steps to minimize those risk factors.

14. Develop daily, monthly, or quarterly routines of internal cleansing and detoxification.

15. Learn about and incorporate ways to boost the strength of your immune system.

16. Reduce the amount of stress in your life.

17. Get plenty of rest.

18. Take a good multivitamin and mineral formula daily, combined with a separate multiple antioxidant and phytonutrient formula.

19. Consider becoming a vegetarian. Consider the attributes of macrobiotics. Establish a dietary program that is geared toward the prevention of all types of cancer.

20. Incorporate soy products into your daily dietary regimen.

21. Maintain a positive attitude, in sickness and in health.

22. Supplement with enzymes daily, preferably a multiple enzyme formula.

23. Eliminate milk and replace it with soymilk.

24. Have yearly digital rectal exams if you are over forty. PSA (prostate-specific antigen) levels should also be checked every year after age fifty.

25. Eat a tomato or some tomato-based products every day.

It is imperative that before devising or changing any existing plan of action, medication or prescribed routine you check with your healthcare professional.

ONE SIZE DOES NOT FIT ALL

One plan does not fit all, and no plan geared toward prevention is written in stone. This means that you can change, add to, or delete things from your plan as your needs change. While my 25 Point Plan can get you started, there are many more preventive measures or things you can do to save your prostate gland. In fact, I've come up with seventy—most of which have been mentioned in this book; but there are probably lots more.

70 WAYS TO SAVE YOUR PROSTATE GLAND

1. Take a variety of antioxidants.
2. Reduce your saturated fat intake. Give up fried foods. Bake or broil them instead.
3. Supplement your diet with fatty acids. Make essential fatty acids, especially flaxseed oil, a daily part of your dietary or supplementary regimen.
4. Stop or don't start smoking.
5. Reduce intake of alcoholic beverages (especially beer).
6. Limit exposure to pesticides and other environmental contaminants, such as lead and cadmium.
7. Keep cholesterol levels below 200 mg per deciliter of blood. Check your cholesterol and triglyceride levels semiannually for elevation.
8. Maintain acceptable fiber intake (30–50 grams daily).
9. Reduce stressful episodes.
10. Have yearly digital rectal exams.
11. Consume generous helpings of fresh fruits and vegetables.
12. Lose excess weight.
13. Consider the attributes of "seed implantation" if prostate cancer is diagnosed.
14. Reduce your intake of milk and dairy products.
15. Eat generous portions of soy products. Learn to love foods made from soy.
16. Reduce or eliminate red meat from your diet. Eat more fish and chicken instead.
17. Eat one cup of pumpkin seeds daily.

18. Supplement your diet with zinc (30–50 mg a day). Check with your health care provider.
19. Supplement your diet with herbs like saw palmetto, pygeum, and others.
20. Practice daily detox methods.
21. Keep your colon clean.
22. Consider attributes of short to medium range fasting.
23. Utilize hydrotherapy if necessary to increase circulation to the prostate gland. Take sitz bats.
24. Take a multiple vitamin and mineral formula daily.
25. Use digestive enzymes.
26. Don't ignore symptoms of BPH.
27. Ask questions. Talk, learn, discuss, educate yourself and others.
28. Limit exposure to x-rays and various biomagnetic fields.
29. Reduce daily caloric intake (especially if you're in the 2,600–3,000 range).
30. Drink clean fresh water (eight glasses a day).
31. Increase vitamin C intake (3,000–5,000 mg daily) with bioflavonoids.
32. Choose anti-cancer foods. For instance, learn to love tomatoes.
33. Add garlic to your diet. Supplement your daily multiple vitamin with garlic extracts and/or capsules.
34. Reduce or avoid use of decongestants and antihistamines.
35. Eat more complex carbohydrates.
36. Check your home water supplies periodically for contamination, especially in cases of non-monitoring by a municipality.
37. After age forty, have yearly exams of the stool to detect microscopic traces of blood.
38. Don't smoke and drink (alcohol) at the same time.

39. Get plenty of sleep.

40. Exercise, exercise, exercise. Take daily walks. Don't become a couch potato.

41. Consider becoming a vegetarian.

42. Develop a healthy sexual relationship with your partner.

43. Eat a carrot every day.

44. Substitute green tea for your coffee.

45. Consume cranberry juice four or five times a week.

46. Use cold pressed oil, such as olive and safflower. Cook with olive oil.

47. Maintain a complementary level of herbs that support or enhance immune function.

48. Break the code of silence.

49. Use chemical-free household cleaning products.

50. Do not use tanning parlors.

51. Know your heredity susceptibility.

52. Abstain from on and off withholding of ejaculate during sexual intercourse, as this causes undue stress to the prostate gland.

53. Do not take supplemental iron above current RDA (10 mgs) unless specified by your doctor.

54. Consider the attributes of drinking gingko tea.

55. Drink fresh vegetable juices.

56. Maintain a regular regimen of products like acidophilus that help maintain levels of friendly intestinal bacteria.

57. Adhere to nature's call—don't suppress the need to urinate.

58. You are not a victim of prostate dysfunction. Practice prevention!

59. Read labels. Use products free from artificial colors, flavorings or harmful chemicals.

60. Take lycopene (tomato) supplements.

61. Consider the attributes of supplemental DHEA or 7-Keto-DHEA.

62. Spend some time in the sunshine to increase your exposure to ultraviolet light and the natural manufacture of vitamin D.

63. Get a second opinion if serious medical–surgical options are needed. Know all your options in cases of medical intervention.

64. Become a "green giant," utilizing chlorophyll, chlorella, blue-green algae and other cellular mediators.

65. Limit extensive bike or horseback rides.

66. Limit use of white flour, sugars, and salt. Consider using honey or fructose instead of sugar substitutes, as they are known carcinogens.

67. Take selenium supplements daily.

68. Take vitamin E daily (400 IUs).

69. Avoid spicy foods.

70. Make sure your home gets adequate ventilation.

In this chapter I have outlined some key programs and protocols aimed at prevention of prostate disease and the management and maintenance of the prostate gland. These protocols also are aimed at and can be used by individuals battling their way back to health. If there is any one thing you learn from this book, please remember, your body has the capability to defend and repair itself at the same time when supplied with the right tools to do so.

This you can control!

Chronological aging is immaterial if you maintain a healthy lifestyle. Don't wait to get started. You should begin to put into action what you have learned, and be prepared to make changes to that plan as the situation dictates. You need to take the same proactive approach that many males have when it comes to their automobiles. For example:

- ◆ You do not wait until your car runs low on oil before putting more oil in.

- ◆ You do not wait until it is twenty degrees below zero to put antifreeze in your car.

- ◆ You do not wait until the oil in your car has turned to sludge before changing it.

- ◆ You do not wait to check or change worn or frail radiator belts and hoses.

- ◆ You do not wait until you've reached 100,000 miles on your car before having it tuned up.

Any of you who personally takes care of his automobile, and those of you who don't but have regular service check-ups or monthly or quarterly maintenance, know the importance these checkups have to the life of your vehicle. You care for your car because you are experientially familiar with the second law of thermodynamics, which states that any system left to itself will undergo entropy. All systems in our universe are linked to this fundamental law of the order of nature.

All living things break down over time. You should not wait until your prostate gland and its proper metabolic functions begin to run down before taking charge and planning a course of action that is designed to maintain health. An aggressive plan of prevention appears to be the key to offset the natural entropy of this small but important gland.

The next chapter, "Getting The Help You Need," will put you in touch with a number of organizations, health centers, hospitals, and web sites in the U.S. and around the world. It will also help you move from the thinking and planning stage to the action phase, which will improve your health.

Please read on!

CHAPTER NINE

GETTING THE
HELP YOU NEED

Most of the people whose experiences I have related heard dis-
couraging words from health professionals, especially from
medical doctors who told them there was no hope, nothing more
to be done, and no possibility of getting better. They did not buy
it. Instead they never gave up hope that there was help to be
found somewhere.

—Andrew Weil, M.D.

As Dr. Weil reports, the most successful patients—those who
tend to recover from serious illnesses—actively search out pos-
sibilities for treatments and cures and follow up every lead they
come across. They ask questions, read books and articles, go
to libraries, write to authors, talk to friends for ideas, and
search for help or meet with different practitioners.

I consider myself one of those successful patients. My illness
changed my life! In my pursuit of optimal health, I have gained
the knowledge to cultivate and manage that treasure—my re-
gained health.

To gain control and manage your prostate disturbances
while preventing further complications, your best defense is to
view your impending problems as an opportunity to make the
necessary changes to regain and preserve your health.

While I consider my case and the consequent recovery and rediscovery of my role in maintaining and managing my own health monumental, another case that serves as a remarkable example of not buying into the notion that there is nothing more to do is that of Anthony J. Sattilaro, a prominent medical doctor. Sattilaro's journey back to health became a best selling book, titled *Recalled By Life.* The most astonishing aspect of this case was the fact that this medical doctor stepped out of a conventional system of healing, which had been his own profession, and into an alternative one.

BREAKING THROUGH TO THE OTHER SIDE

In June of 1978, Dr. Sattilaro, chief executive officer of Methodist Hospital in Philadelphia, was diagnosed with prostate cancer (stage IV D). The cancer had metastasized to other parts of his body. About his approach to treatment Sattilaro wrote:

> Within weeks after the diagnosis was made I underwent surgery and began estrogen treatment to combat the spread of the disease. It soon become apparent, however, that this would not halt the malignancy, and in light of this I began to seek alternatives that might rescue me from death.
> I had been a doctor for more than 20 years by then, and it was no small trepidation that I went looking for answers outside the profession to which I dedicated my life. (p. 1)

Among the alternatives investigated, Sattilaro took up a macrobiotic diet, a Japanese diet regimen that has been reported to reduce the risk of contracting cancer. Despite the fact that this chosen treatment seemed to benefit him, his colleagues' views of his move toward alternative methods was not positive. Most of his peers in the medical profession judged alternative therapies as fraudulent, and said that by involving himself in this mode of treatment he was encouraging other patients to use a system that could be dangerous. Secondly, they argued that although he was getting some miraculous results from his new protocol, mere anecdotal evidence (even his own story), would not be accepted as valid proof of anything.

Dr. Sattilaro eventually died of prostate cancer eleven years after he was first diagnosed in 1978. When he wrote his book in 1982, outlining his incredible journey back to health, the prostate cancer which his colleagues had informed him would take his life in a couple of years was in remission.

Dr. Sattilaro stated that in treating his own cancer, he "put the holistic view of health to the ultimate test," and it saved his life. To his skeptical observers, Sattilaro maintained that if the macrobiotic diet was not responsible for his recovery, then it definitely played a major role in extending his life and improving the quality of his remaining years.

THE LESSONS OF ILLNESS

Despite the invaluable lessons that illness affords, earlier intervention will prevent you from having to learn such lessons through prostate disease. Dr. Robert Sorge, Naturopathic Doctor of the Year in 1978, reminds us that "today's major diseases are degenerative in nature. These conditions can take ten, twenty, thirty years to develop." Sorge maintains that many of these diseases could have been prevented with a nutritional wellness program in advance of the condition. (p. 7)

It took a serious prostate dysfunction for Dr. Sattilaro to come to the realization that the key to maintaining one's life-long health potential is prevention of disease. In essence, it is your individual responsibility to remove "the obstacle to cure." (Whitaker, pp. 3–25)

THE OBSTACLE REMOVED

Dr. Sattilaro had the wisdom and courage to move beyond the prevailing paradigm of his profession. The courage to make such a step is summed up by Gary Null, Ph.D., a notable author and alternative healthcare practitioner. His comments debunk the notion of a massive shift in human consciousness, placing individual responsibility as the determining factor in meaningful change.

To the contrary, today, and throughout world history, you cannot find a single paradigm shift where awareness of what was wrong, and a need or desire to change it, were motivating factors in its transformation...We have never in world history—in our culture or any other—ever had a massive shift in consciousness.

Things don't change, only those people who have the courage to step out of their belief system into another one, change. (pp. 11–12)

The focus of the rest of this book is to put you in touch with individuals, organizations, and treatment centers, both conventional and nonconventional, that will assist you in your quest to step out and change. In the Holistic Health Directory that follows, you will find names, addresses, and telephone numbers of many well-known conventional cancer treatment centers and organizations, as well as alternative and holistic health treatment centers and organizations. You will also find cancer hotlines and websites and a list of suggested reading.

Everything begins and ends with *you* making the commitment to regain your health, and doing the things necessary to maintain it, as Dr. Sattilaro and many others have done. Once the obstacle to cure are removed—life-negative dietary habits, lifestyle factors and belief systems—our chances of maximizing the positive effects of and treatment are greatly enhanced.

The force responsible for healing is within the patient.
—*Deepak Chopra, M.D.*

Good luck, and as always,

Good health to you!

The Holistic Health Directory

Note: Every effort has been made to insure the accuracy of each listing. Please be aware that telephone numbers and addresses are subject to change.

— CONVENTIONAL TREATMENT CENTERS — AND ORGANIZATIONS

TREATMENT CENTERS

While there are many well-known prostate treatment centers in the U.S., the Memorial Sloan-Kettering Cancer Center in New York has a worldwide reputation as one of the best. Others in the U.S. known for innovation and high success rates are:

- Duke University Medical Center, Durham, North Carolina
- Methodist Hospital, Houston, Texas
- Hospital of the University of Pennsylvania, Philadelphia, Pennsylvania
- The Fox Chase Cancer Center, Philadelphia, Pennsylvania
- Johns Hopkins, Baltimore, Maryland
- The Mayo Clinic, Rochester, Minnesota
- Massachusetts General Hospital, Boston, Massachusetts
- UCLA Medical Center, Los Angeles, California

The Hill Burton Free Hospital Program

This is a U.S. federally funded program that provides free hospital care to individuals who qualify. To find out if you qualify, and for a listing of hospitals that participate in this program in your state please call 1-800-638-0742.

ORGANIZATIONS

American Cancer Society
1599 Clifton Road, NE
Atlanta, GA 30329
800-227-2343

American Urological Association
1120 North Charles Street
Baltimore, MD 21201
410-223-4310

Can Survive
6500 Wilshire Boulevard
Los Angeles, CA 90048
310-203-9232

Committee For Freedom of Choice in Medicine, Inc.
1180 Walnut Avenue
Chula Vista, CA 91911
619-429-8200

Foundation of Advancement in Cancer Therapy
P.O. Box 1242
Old Chelsea Station
New York, NY 10113
212-741-2790

International Association of Cancer Victors and Friends
7740 West Manchester Avenue, Ste 110
Playa del Rey, CA 90293
213-822-5032

International Society for Preventive Oncology
217 East 85th Street, Ste 303
New York, NY 10028
212-534-4991

Latin American Cancer Research Project
525 Twenty Third Street, NW
Washington, DC 20037
202-861-3200

Man to Man
c/o American Cancer Society
1599 Clifton Road, NE
Atlanta, GA 30329
800-227-2345

National Cancer Institute
Cancer Information Services
Public Inquiries, Office of Cancer Communication
9000 Rockville Pike
Bethesda, MD 20892
800-4-CANCER

National Cancer Institute
National Institute of Health
Building 21, Room 10A24
Bethesda, MD 20892
800-422-6237

National Coalition for Cancer Survivorship
1010 Wayne Avenue, 5th floor
Silver Springs, MD 20910
301-650-8868

National Kidney and Urologic Disease Information
Clearing House
Box NKUDIC
9000 Rockville Pike
Bethesda, MD 20892
301-468-6345

National Prostate Cancer Coalition

P.O. Box 354
Baltimore, MD 21203-0554
800-242-2383

Patient Advocates for Advanced Cancer Treatments

1143 Parmelee, NW
Grand Rapids, MI 49504
616-453-1477

People Against Cancer

Box 10
Otho, IA 50569
515-972-4444

People's Medical Society

462 Walnut Street
Allentown, PA 18102
215-770-1670

The Wellness Community

2716 Ocean Park Boulevard, Ste 1040
Santa Monica, CA 90404-5211
310-314-2555

American Foundation for Urologic Disease

300 W. Pratt, Ste 401
Baltimore, MD 21201
800-242-2383

Prostate Cancer Communication Resource Inc.

P.O. Box 6023
Carefree, AZ 85377
602-488-1915

Prostate Health Program of New York

785 Park Avenue
New York, NY 10021
212-988-8888

WEB SITES

The Internet is fast becoming a primary source for self-education about all aspects of health. With a little searching, you can discover a treasury of information about prostate cancer and treatment options. Listed below are a few valuable sites to get you started.

National Cancer Institute
  http://www.nci.nih.gov/

Center for Disease and Prevention
  http://www.cdc.gov/cdc.htm/

National Institute of Health
  http://www.nih.gov/

The National Library of Medicine's MEDLINE
  http://www.igm.nim.nih.gov/

Prostate Cancer Infolink
  http://www.comed.com/Prostate/

HOTLINES

Cancer Fax
  301-402-5874
  Note: By using this fax number you can get-up-to-date information about prostate and other cancers from the National Cancer Institute. Entering the corresponding numbers requested, information can be faxed to you immediately.

Cancer Hotline
  816-932-8453

Cancer Information Services (CIS)
  800-422-6237

Fox Chase Cancer Center, Prostate Cancer Hotline
  215-728-2406

Make Today Count
800-432-2273

National Institute of Health
800-4-CANCER

Prostate Cancer Support Network
410-727-2908

Prostate Information Hotline
800-543-9632

— ALTERNATIVE TREATMENT CENTERS — AND ORGANIZATIONS

TREATMENT CENTERS

American Academy of Environmental Medicine
4510 West 89th Street, Ste 110
Prairie Village, KS 66207-2282
913-642-6062

American Whole Health Clinic Inc.
Lincoln Park Center
990 West Fullerton Avenue, Ste 300
Chicago, IL 60614
773-296-6700

Cancer Care Center for Integrated Treatment and Research
521 Hammill Lane
Reno, NV 89509
702-827-0707

Cancer Treatment Centers of America
3455 Salt Creek Lane, Ste 200
Arlington Heights, IL 60005-1090
800-955-2822

Center for Holistic Medicine and Ayurveda

6366 Sherwood Road
Philadelphia, PA 19151
or
330 Breezewood Road
Lehighton, PA 18235
215-473-4226
215-473-7453

Center For Integrative Medicine
Thomas Jefferson University Hospital

Ford Road Campus
Park Plaza Condominiums
3900 Ford Road, Ste B
Philadelphia, PA 19131
800-JEFF-NOW or
215-879-5121

Complementary and Alternative Medicine at the NIH

Office of Alternative Medicine Clearing House
P.O. Box 8218
Silver Springs, MD 20907-8218
888-644-6226

Gerson Institute

P.O. Box 430
Bonita, CA 91908
888-4-GERSON

Hospital Santa Monica

870 Canarios Court
Chula Vista, CA (no zip here)
800-359-6547

King County Natural Medicine Clinic

(In Association with Bastyr University and Community Health
Centers of King County)
8309 South 259th Street
Kent, WA 98031
253-852-2866

Livingston Foundation Medical Center
3239 Duke Street
San Diego, CA 92110
888-777-7321 (US and Canada)

Magaziner Medical Center
1907 Greentree Road
Cherry Hill, NJ 08034
800-424-8222

The Atkins Center for Complementary Medicine
152 East 55th Street
New York, NY 10022
212-758-2110

The Integrative Medicine Clinic
The University of Arizona College of Medicine
P.O. Box 245153
Tucson, AZ 85724-5153
520-694-6555

The Kuhnau Center, Tijuana B.C. Mexico
U.S. mailing address:
P.O. Box 432014
San Ysidro, CA 92143
(Specializes in embryonic shark tissue transplants)

The Perlmutter Health Center
800 Goodlette Road North, Ste 270
Naples, FL, 34102
941-649-7400

The Raj Maharishi–Ayur–Veda Clinic
1734 Jasmine Avenue
Fairfield, Iowa 52556
800-248-9050

The Shealy Institute for Comprehensive Medicine
1328 East Evergreen
Springfield, MO 65803
417-865-5940

The Village at Newtown Medical Center
2700 S. Eagle Road
Newtown, PA 18940-1570
215-579-1300

Valley Cancer Institute
12099 West Washington Boulevard, Ste 304
Los Angeles, CA 90066
800-488-1370 or 213-398-0013

ORGANIZATIONS

American Association of Alternative Healers
P.O. Box 10026
Sedona, AZ 86335-8026

American Association of Naturopathic Physicians
2366 Eastlake Avenue, East, Ste 322
Seattle, WA 98102
206-323-7610

American Botanical Council
P.O. Box 20166
Austin, TX 78720-1660
512-331-8868

American Holistic Medical Association
4101 Lake Boone Trail, Ste 201
Raleigh, NC 27067

American Preventive Medical Association
459 Walker Road
Great Falls, VA 22066
703-759-0662

Association of Natural Medicine Pharmacists
1 Espaloa Court
San Rafael, CA 94901
415-453-3534

Biofeedback Certification Institute of America
10200 West 44th Avenue, Ste 304
Wheat Ridge, CO 80033-2840
303-420-2902

Cancer Control Society
2043 North Berendo
Los Angeles, CA 90027

Herb Research Foundation
1007 Pearl Street, Ste 200
Boulder, CO 80302
800-748-2617

Holistic Health Association of Princeton New Jersey
366 Nassau Street
Princeton, NJ 08540
609-924-3836

International Academy of Nutrition
P.O. Box 18433
Asheville, NC 28814
704-258-3243

International Association of Colon Hydrotherapy
12204 Northwest, Loop 410
San Antonio, TX 78230
210-366-2888

International Society for the Study of Subtle Energies and Energy Medicine
356 Coldeo Circle
Golden, CO 80403
303-278-2288

Macrobiotic Medicine/Kushi Institute
P.O. Box 7
Becket, MA 01223
413-623-5741

National Center for Homeopathy
801 North Fairfax Street, Ste 306
Alexandria, VA 22314

Northwest Coalition for Alternatives to Pesticides
P.O. Box 1393
Eugene, OR 97440
503-344-5044

The Ayurvedic Institute
P.O. Box 2345
Albuquerque, NM 87192-1445
505-291-9698

Tri-State Holistic Health Association
P.O. Box 1581
Voorhees, NJ 08043
609-755-1155

WEB SITES

Alternative Medicine
http://www.alternativemedicine.com

Health World Online
http://www.healthy.net

University of Texas Center for Alternative Medicine Research in Cancer (UTCAM)
http://www.sph.uth.tmc.edu/utcam

National Institute of Ayurvedic Medicine
http://www.niam.com

Office of Alternative Medicine
http://www.altmed.od.nih.gov/

Q and A with a Holistic Doctor
http://www.tripod.com/health/

HOTLINES

**Complementary and Alternative Medicine
at National Institute of Health**
888-644-6226

Contre Cancer Care Center
800-500-HOPE

Delaware Valley Wellness Network
610-355-2300 or 215-477-1944

Holistic Health Referral Service
(serves the Philadelphia and New Jersey areas)
610-407-9100 or 215-477-1944

Natural Library of Medicine
301-496-6308

Physicians for Alternative Medicine
800-717-5649

The MD's Holistic Health Line
900-GET-WELL

World Research Foundation
818-999-5483
Note: Will send packet of information of many different non-conventional treatment protocols for specified condition.

— THE INTERNATIONAL —
CONNECTION

The list that follows gives an overview of some well-known clinics, organizations and treatment centers around the globe. Many of these centers practice conventional as well as non-conventional treatment. Additionally, many of these centers are using therapies which have not been approved for use in the United States, but have a record of success based on scientific trials and their application.

TREATMENT CENTERS AND ASSOCIATIONS

American Biologics—Mexico
Hospital and Integrative Medical Center
Tijuana, B.C., Mexico
800-785-0490
Note: Most American private insurance companies reimburse patients for most therapies offered at this institute according to American Biologics.

American Association of Orthomolecular Medicine
7375 Kingsway
Burnaby, BC, V3N3B5, Canada

African Organization for Research and Training in Cancer
University of Zimbabwe
P.O.Box A178
Zimbabwe, Africa

Bircher–Benner Privat Klinik
Kelltnesstasse 48
CH 8044 Zurich, Switzerland
(011) 41-1251-68-90

Canadian Cancer Society
10 Alcorn Avenue, Ste 200
Toronto Ontario, Canada, M4V3B1
416-961-7223

Cancer Information and Support Society
39 Atchison Street
Stileonards
New South Wales 2065, Australia
(02) 906-2189

Center for Cell Specific Cancer Therapy
Dominican Republic
www.csct.com
877-741-2728 (Toll Free)

**Certified Therapy Center
IAT Clinic—Immunology Research Center**
  Freeport, Bahamas
  242-352-7555

Cheltenham Cancer Help Centre
  14 Clarence Square
  Cheltenham, Gloucestershire GL 504JN, England
  (011) 44-242-525437

Chiltern Cancer Counseling
  193 Tring Road. Aylesbury
  Buckinghamshire HP201JH, England
  (0296) 24854

Chronic Disease Control and Treatment Center
  Am Reuthlein
  D-8675 Bad Steben, Germany
  011-49-9288/ 5161

E.D. Danopoulou, M.D.
  Rigillis Street 26
  Holistic Medical Clinic
  1-18-11 KY Building 6F
  Kita Oostsuka, Toshima-Ku
  Tokyo 170, Japan
  03-3940-8071

**European Association for Cancer Research
Cancer Research Campaign Labs**
  University of Nottingham
  Nottingham NG72RD, United Kingdom
  Phone (44602)48 48 48 ext. 3401

**European Organization for Cooperation in Cancer
Prevention Studies**
  Avenue R Vandendnessche, B-1150
  Bruxelles, Belgium
  (322) 762-0485

European Society for Cancer, Internal/Medicine
Centre Antoine Lacassagne
36 Vole Romaine
F-06054 Nice, France

Hans A. Nieper, M.D.
Sedan Strasse 21
3000 Hanover 1, Germany
011-49-511-348-0808
Note: Dr. Nieper served as president of the German Society
of Oncology from 1982 to 1985.

Immuno-Argumentative Therapy
P.O. Box F-2689
Freeport, Grand Bahama Island,
Bahamas
(809) 352-7455/6

International Medical Center
16 de Septembre #2215
3202 CD Juarez, Mexico
0115216-16-26-01

International Union Against Cancer
Rue du Consell General 3, CH-1205
Geneva, Switzerland
(41 22) 720 18 11

Itotaka Yo Joen Holistic Health Center
7528-20 Ariake Hotaka-Cho
Minamiazumi-Gun
Nagano Prefecture 399-83, Japan
(0263) 83-5260

Meditation for Cancer Patients
50 Garnet Street
Dulwhich Hill, New South Wales 2203,
Australia
(02)559-5666

Middle East Federation Against Cancer
Cancer Institute
174 Tahrir Street
Cairo, Egypt

New Approaches to Cancer
5 Larksfield; Egham
Surrey, TW 20 ORB
United Kingdom
(0784) 433610

Radiant Health Centre
Doctors Hill/Goomalling Road
West Australia 6401
(096) 22 346

Schafer's Health Centre Ltd.
Box 251, Unity, Saskatchewan
S0K 4LO, Canada
306-228-2512

— SUGGESTED READING —

Note: Recommended reading about nutrition and cancer is found in Chapter Seven.

Dixon, B.M., *Good Health For African Americans,* New York, NY: Crown Publishers, Inc., 1994.

Evans, R.A., *Making the Right Choice, Treatment Options in Cancer Surgery,* Garden City Park, NY: Avery Publishing Group, 1995.

Farquhar, J.W., *The American Way of Life Need Not be Hazardous to Your Health,* Reading, Massachusetts: Addison-Wesley, 1987.

King, D., J. King, and J. Pearlroth, *Cancer Combat,* New York, NY: Bantam Books, 1998.

Konner, M., *Medicine at the Crossroads, The Crisis in Health Care,* New York: Pantheon Books,1993.

Kushi, A., and A. Jack, *Complete Guide to Macrobiotic Cooking,* New York: Warner Books, 1985.

Levenstein, M.K., *Everyday Cancer Risks and How to Avoid Them,* Garden City Park, NY: Avery Publishing Group, 1982.

Mackarness, J.R., *Living Safely in a Polluted World,* New York: Stein and Day Publishers, 1980.

Morter, T., *Your Health, Your Choice,* Hollywood, Fla: Lifetime Books, Inc., 1995.

Moss, R.W., *Cancer Therapy: The Independent Consumer's Guide to Non-Toxic Treatment and Prevention,* Brooklyn, NY: Equinox Press. Inc., 1992.

Oesterling, J.E., and M.A. Moyad, *The ABC's of Prostate Cancer,* Lanham, Maryland: Madison Books, 1997.

Pauling. L., *How to Live Longer and Feel Better,* New York: Freeman and Company, 1986.

Preuss, H.G., B. Adderly, *The Prostate Cure,* New York: Crown Publishing Inc., 1998.

Reed, J.W., N. B. Shulman, and C. Shucker, *The Black Man's Guide to Good Health,* New York: The Berkeley Publishing Group, 1994.

Sattilaro, A.J., *Recalled By Life,* Boston: Houghton Mifflin Co., 1982.

Weil, A., *Spontaneous Healing,* New York: Fawcett Columbine, 1995.

KNOW YOUR PROSTATE CANCER RISK FACTOR

SELF–TEST FOR PROSTATE CANCER RISK

This test measures your risk of developing prostate cancer. Circle the score for each characteristic that applies to you. Total the score, then check your risk category on the next page.

Family History
Choose any that apply.

+2 Your father, uncle or brother had prostate cancer

+3 More than one close relative had prostate cancer

+1 You are black

–2 You are oriental

Diet
Choose any that apply.

+3 You eat whole-milk dairy products, such as cheese, butter, cream cheese and whole milk, every day or almost everyday

+2 You eat fried or butter-sauce foods several times a week

+2 You eat pastries, ice cream or rich desserts at least several times a week

+2 You eat fatty meats, such as steak, hamburger, roast beef, sausage or cold cuts, almost every day

+2 You eat lots of butter, margarine or fried foods almost every day

+2 You eat high-fat, empty-calorie foods, such as chips, dips or French fries, several times a week

Personal
Choose any that apply.

+5 You took, or are taking, testosterone or androgen medication

+2 You are overweight by 20%

+3 You are overweight by more than 25%

INTERPRETING YOUR SCORE

To determine your score, add all scores from the categories. Check your total score below to see if your health and your life are at risk.

0–8 **Low Risk**. Your risk of prostate cancer is low, but don't overlook having an annual examination of the prostate gland if you are 40 or older.

9–15 **Moderate Risk.** Your risk of prostate cancer is moderate. Have an annual examination of the prostate gland if you are 40 or older.

16–22 **High Risk.** You are at high risk of developing prostate cancer. Have an examination of your prostate twice a year. Losing weight by following a permanent weight-loss diet will help lower your risk.

23+ **Very High Risk.** You are at very high risk of developing prostate cancer. Have yearly or more-frequent prostate examinations. Lose weight with he permanent weight-loss diet, and follow a risk-reducing nutrition plan to help lower your risk.

Source: Howard, Elliott J., M.D., *Health Risks*, Tucson, Ariz: The Body Press, 1986, pp.76,77. Used with permission.

HOW TO DECIPHER SCIENTIFIC REPORTING

This report will assist you in deciphering and finding answers concerning the efficacy of a protocol when reviewing the scientific data available on it. The science behind treatment, drug approval or how a supplement works can be overwhelming. When one is attempting to make a decision based on the most recent information available, the unfamiliar terminology can make a study appear to be more imposing than it really is.

Whenever you are trying to assess the most up-to-date information you are doing research on, there are several questions you should ask yourself. For example:

1. Were people studied or rodents?
2. How good are these numbers?
3. Who paid for the study?
4. Were researchers looking forward to backward?
5. How were the subjects chosen?
6. What do other health groups say?

In your quest to find answers to your questions, you might use the following guide to test the parameters of a study or information you have heard or have at hand. If you ask yourself the above questions, how well do they stack up against the answers below?

IN SEARCH OF ANSWERS

Who or what was studied?

Sometimes research with humans is neither desirable nor possible. When a study reports, for example, that rice bran lowers blood cholesterol was done with hamsters, in this case, it may be best to make your final judgement when human trials are completed.

What about the numbers?

In general terms, the more subjects (people, places, or things) used in a study and the longer its duration, the more reliable will be the facts and conclusions drawn from this study.

Who paid the tab?

This is important when looking at the efficacy and possible soundness of certain communiques. For example, a study may say," a recent study of oat bran was funded by Quaker Oats on its cholesterol lowering effects." This is not necessarily bad, but a good reason to view other studies done by independent (outside) researchers that have found similar findings when conducting the same test.

Going Forward or Backward?

Researchers believe that the most reliable results are obtained from "prospective" (forthcoming) studies, in which investigators control the food, drug or activity throughout the examination. If a study is "retrospective" (backward or past) the scientists are dependent on reports of past behavior from the subjects themselves. In these cases, information is often cloudy, as exact information may have been forgotten by past participants.

Are the subjects equal?

Scientific investigators consider data from studies to be "suspect" when the experimental group (the one receiving the food, treatment or drug) is not a perfect match for the control group (made up of volunteers who may be more health conscious and motivated—they may not be comparable to a group of non-volunteers).

What's the word on the street?

There is a hoard of information available, which is reported daily in newspapers, magazines, radio, and on the Internet. Many of these studies years ago would have been buried in medical journals. However, mass media can report and whet the appetite of a health-information-hungry society today, even though all the information may not be meaningful.

How do you make sure the "hype" does not overwhelm the science? Stay informed and practice moderation. To make sure you have a clear understanding of some terms that may be unfamiliar please use the following guide.

UNDERSTANDING SCIENTIFIC TERMINOLOGY

Anecdotal (Personal) Testimonials: Research based on casual observation, not rigorous scientific investigation. It may be valid, but isn't proven.

Clinical Study: A study that uses people as its subjects.

Controlled Experiment: A form of research that looks at cause and effect. Researchers here work with groups that are comparable in all aspects, except for treatment being tested. In essence, any differences that occur between the group or thing being tested can be attributed to the treatment.

Double Blind: Neither the subjects nor the investigators have any knowledge of the treatment (product or thing) being used. This type of study is considered to be very reliable, because it deters bias (a predisposed point of view) by the researcher or sponsor.

Experimental Bias: Behavior by researchers that can influence the outcome of a study.

Experimental Data: Information collected during a study.

Experimental Group: The group of subjects that get the active treatments.

Placebo: A substance having no medicinal value that appears identical to the real treatment agent used in a study.

Single Blind: Controlled research in which subjects don't know whether they are receiving the treatment or a placebo.

Variable: The characteristic of an organism, environment, or experimental situation that can vary from one environment to another, or from one experimental situation to another.

In Vitro: A process or reaction carried out in a petri dish or test tube.

In Vivo: A process or reaction carried out in a living organism.

HOW TO CLEANSE THE LIVER & GALLBLADDER

One of the hallmarks of natural medicine is attention to the condition of the internal organs, especially the liver and gallbladder. It is surprisingly easy to use herbs and nutrients to safely and effectively cleanse these organs.

Many holistic practitioners, in fact, recommend such an organ cleansing on a yearly basis as a disease-prevention and health-maintenance strategy. The following liver and gallbladder flush procedure come from Keith DeOrio, M.D., director of the DeOrio Medical Group in Santa Monica, California.

THE FLUSH

The flush, which calls for apple juice or cider, Epsom salts and olive oil, works as a detoxifying agent to restore normal function to the liver and gallbladder, according to Dr. K. DeOrio. The acids in the apple juice help to soften gallstones, the magnesium in the Epsom salts relaxes the sphincters of the gallbladder and bile duct, and the olive oil produces contractions in the liver and gallbladder, which help in the excretion of stored waste materials. To do the flush, Dr. DeOrio typically advises following these steps:

Days 1–5: Follow your usual diet. Drink as much apple juice or cider (preferably organic) as possible on these days, diluting the juice with an equal amount of water. While individual tolerances vary, Dr. DeOrio recommends drinking at least one-half gallon of the diluted juice each day. Add one ounce of Phosfood (a product that helps dissolve gallstones)* to each gallon of juice before it is diluted.

Day 6 (noon): Eat lunch as usual.

Day 6 (3 P.M.): Dissolve two teaspoons of Epsom salts in two ounces of hot water and drink. To offset the unpleasant taste, Dr. DeOrio suggests following this with a little freshly squeezed orange juice.

Day 6 (bedtime): Before bed, moderately heat one-half cup of cold-pressed olive oil and then drink the oil, followed by one-half cup of orange juice. Alternatively, you may blend the olive oil with the juice and drink the mixture. Immediately afterward, get into bed and lie on your right side with your right knee pulled up to your chest. This ensures that the liver, located on the right side of the body at the base of the rib cage, receives the full benefit of the olive oil/orange juice mixture. Maintain this position for thirty minutes, then sleep normally.

Day 7: One hour before breakfast, dissolve two teaspoons of Epsom salts in two ounces of hot water and drink.

Dr. DeOrio cautions that some people experience mild nausea or, in rare cases, vomiting when drinking the olive oil and orange juice mixture. Though momentarily uncomfortable, these symptoms are actually a good sign, confirming that the flush is working. The nausea is due to the release of stored toxins from the gallbladder and liver. Both nausea and vomiting should pass after a few hours, according to Dr. DeOrio.

---

*To find out more about Phosfood, or to purchase Phosfood, contact Standard Process, P.O. Box 1289, Alameda, CA 94501, 1-800-662-9134.

If one experiences pain in the upper right abdomen following flush, Dr. DeOrio usually suggests drinking another two teaspoons of Epsom salts dissolved in hot water. If pain persists for more than four to six hours, consult a physician.

Caution: Consult a qualified health professional before you begin any detoxification program.

Reprinted with permission from *Alternative Medicine* magazine, June/July, 1998, Issue #24, p. 13. 800-333-HEAL *www.alternative medicine.com*

REFERENCES

Opening Quotes

Balch, J. F., and P. A. Balch. *Prescription for Nutritional Healing.* Garden City Park, N.Y.: Avery, 1996.

Fox, A., and B. Fox. *The Healthy Prostate.* New York: John Wiley and Sons, 1996.

Janson, M. quoted in Rynk, P. "A Health Care Guide Especially For Men." *Be Healthy.* (July/Aug 1992): 10.

Rosenfield, I. *The Best Treatment.* New York: Simon and Schuster, 1991.

Preface

Howard, E. T. *Health Risk.* Tucson, Ariz.: The Body Press, 1986.

Preuss, H. G. and B. Adderly. *The Prostate Cure.* New York: Crown, 1998.

Rosenfield, I. *The Best Treatment.* New York: Simon and Schuster, 1991.

Walsh, P. C. and J. Worthington. *The Prostate: A Guide for Men and the Women Who Love Them.* Baltimore: The Johns Hopkins University Press, 1995.

Whitaker, J. Dr. *Whitaker's Guide to Natural Healing.* Rocklin, Calif.: Prima, 1995.

Introduction

Balch, J. F. and P. A. Balch. *Prescription for Nutritional Healing.* Garden City Park, N.Y.: Avery, 1996.

Eisenberg, D. M. "Trends in Alternative Medicine Use in the United States, 1990–1997." *Journal of the American Medical Association,* (Nov. 11, 1998) 280 (18): 1569–1575.

Eisenberg, D. M. et al. "Unconventional Medicine in the United States." *The New England Journal of Medicine.* 328 (1993): 246–52.

Fredericks, C. *Nutritional Guide for the Prevention and Cure of Common Ailments and Diseases.* New York: Simon and Schuster, 1982.

"The Politics of Medicine: 31% of Americans left out in the cold, despite $1 trillion for U.S. health care." *Alternative Medicine Digest,* no. 16 (1997): 82–83.

Chapter One

Bieler, H. G. and S. Nichols. *Dr. Bieler's Natural Way to Sexual Health.* Los Angeles: Charles Publishing, 1972.

Colgan, M. *Your Vitamin Profile.* New York: Quill, 1982, p. 70.

Editors of Prevention Magazine. *Twelve Modern Medical Miracles for Men Only.* Emmaus, Penn.: Rodale Press, 1989, pp. 41–43.

Fox, A. and B. Fox. *The Healthy Prostate.* New York: John Wiley and Sons, 1996.

Howard, E. J. *Health Risk.* Tucson: The Body Press, 1986.

"Keeping Your Prostate Healthy with Natural Remedies." *Alternative Medicine Digest,* (March 1999): 50–52.

King, B. C. and M. J. Showers. *Human Anatomy and Physiology.* Philadelphia: W.B. Saunders, 1969.

Memmler, R. H. et al. *The Human Body in Health and Disease.* Philadelphia: Lippincott, 1996.

Preuss, H. G. and B. Adderly. *The Prostate Cure.* New York: Crown, 1998.

Ratcliff, J. D. *Your Body and How It Works.* Pleasantville, N.Y.: Reader's Digest Press, 1975.

Scher, H. "Prostate Cancer: Where Do We Go From Here?" *Current Opinion in Oncology 3* (1991): 568–574.

Wallner, K. *Prostate Cancer: A Non-Surgical Perspective.* New York: Smart Medicine, 1996.

Walsh, P. C. and J. Worthington. *The Prostate: A Guide for Men and the Women Who Love Them.* Baltimore: The Johns Hopkins University Press, 1995.

Weil, A. *8 Weeks to Optimum Health.* New York: Alfred A. Knopf, 1997.

———. *Spontaneous Healing.* New York: Fawcett Columbine, 1995.

Chapter Two

Berger, S. *Forever Young.* New York: William Morrow, 1989.

Bostwick, D. G. and C. T. Maclennan. *Prostate Cancer: What Every Man and His Family Needs to Know.* New York: Villard, 1996.

Colgan, M. *Your Personal Vitamin Profile.* New York: Quill, 1982.

Dolby Toews, V. "8 Cellular Bodyguards for Your Health." *Better Nutrition,* (May 1999): 36–42.

Gelbard, M. *Solving Prostate Problems.* New York: Simon and Schuster, 1995.

Gittleman, A. L. *Super Nutrition for Men and the Women Who Love Them.* New York: M. Evans and Company, 1996.

Hoffman, M. and W. LeGro. *Disease Free.* Emmaus, Penn.: Rodale, 1993.

"Men's Health Alert." *Community Service Bulletin,* Fox Chase Cancer Center, Philadelphia, Pa. (Mar 1999).

Miller, B. A. (editor-in-chief). *Racial/Ethnic Patterns of Cancer in the United States.* Bethesda, Md., SEER Program, National Institutes of Health, National Cancer Institute, Publication no. 98-4104 (May 1998): 109–111.

National Cancer Institute. *Spread the Word About Cancer: A Guide for Black Americans.* Bethesda, Md.: National Institutes of Health, Publication no. 96-3412 (1995): 4–8.

National Cancer Institute. *Understanding Prostate Changes: A Health Guide for All Men.* Bethesda, Md.: National Institutes of Health, Publication no. 98-4303 (Sept 1998): 14.

National Cancer Institute. *When Canser Recurs: Meeting the Challenge Again.* Bethesda, MD: National Institutes of Health, Publication no. 93-2709 (Oct. 1992): 16–20.

Osterling, J.E. and M.A. Moyad, *The ABC's of Prostate Cancer,* Lanham, MD, 199x.

Prostate Health, Without Drugs or Surgury. Toronto: Life Force Laboratories, 1999.

Salmans, S. *Prostate Questions You Have . . . Answers You Need.* Allentown, Penn.: People's Medical Society, 1993.

Theodosakis, J.; B. Adderly; and B. Fox. *The Arthritis Cure.* New York: St Martin's, 1997.

Waldron, C. "Black Men Push for More Funding, Education for Prostate Cancer." *Jet Magazine,* (Feb. 2, 19988: 24–25.

Walsh, P. C. and H. Farrer. *The Prostate: A Guide for Men and The Women Who Love Them,* Baltimore: The Johns Hopkins University Press, 1995.

Chapter Three

Atkins, R. C. *Dr. Atkins' Vita Nutrient Solution.* New York: Simon and Schuster, 1998.

Fox, A. and B. Fox. *The Healthy Prostate.* New York: John Wiley, 1996, p. 29.

Gelband, M. and W. Bentley. *Solving Prostate Problems.* New York: Simon and Schuster, 1995.

Goldstein, J. A. *Could Your Doctor Be Wrong?* New York: Pharos, 1991.

Kaltenbach, D. *How to Interpret Your Biopsy and Other Lab Reports.* New Port Richey: Fl.: Prostate Cancer Research Network, 1994.

Wallner, K. *Prostate Cancer: A Non-Surgical Perspective.* Canaan, N.Y.: Smart Medicine, 1996.

Walsh, P. C. and J. Worthington. *The Prostate: A Guide for Men and the Women Who Love Them.* Baltimore: The Johns Hopkins University Press, 1995.

Chapter Four

Arky, R. and C. S. Davison. *Physicians' Desk Reference.* 51st ed. Montvale, N.J.: Medical Economics Company, 1997.

Meyer, S. and S. C. Nash. *Prostate Cancer: Making Survival Decisions.* Chicago: The University of Chicago Press, 1994.

Murray, M. T. and J. Pizzorno. *Encyclopedia of Natural Medicine.* Rocklin, Calif.: Prima, 1991.

National Cancer Institute. *When Cancer Recurs: Meeting the Challenge Again.* Bethesda, Md.: National Institutes of Health, Publication no. 93-2709 (Oct. 1992): 16–20.

Salmans, S. *Prostate Questions You Have . . . Answers You Need.* Allentown, Penn.: People's Medical Society, 1993.

Wallner, K. *Prostate Cancer: A Non-Surgical Perspective.* New York: Smart Medicine, 1996, p. 1.

Chapter Five

Airola, P. *How to Get Well.* Sherwood, Oreg.: Health Plus, 1989.

Ballentine, R. "The Healing Force of Energy." *Let's Live Magazine* 67, no. 3 (March 1999): 80.

Borysenko, J. *Minding the Body, Mending the Mind.* Reading, Mass., Addison Wesley, 1987.

Borysenko, J. *Fire in the Soul.* New York: Warmer Books, 1983.

Burke, E. "Aerobics for Prostate Health." *Nutritional Insights, Your Natural Health Navigator* (Supplement to *Let's Live*) 2, no. 7 (July 1997): 24.

Cheraskin, E.; W. M. Ringsdorf et al. *Diet and Disease.* New Canaan, Conn.: Keats, 1987.

Chopra, D. "One More Reality to Go." *Inner Realm Magazine* 2, no. 4 (April 1999): 6–8.

Crayhon, R. *Health Benefits of FOS (Fructoligosaccharides).* New Canaan, Conn.: Keats, 1995.

DeOrio, K. "How to Do a Liver and Gallbladder Clean-Out." *Alternative Medicine Digest* 24 (June/July 1998): 13.

Donsbach, K. W. *Cancer: Allopathic and Wholistic Therapy, a Comparison.* Rosarito Beach, Mexico: Hospital Santa Monica, 1999.

Donsbach, K. W. and H. R. Alseben. *Wholistic Cancer Therapy.* Tulsa, Okla.: The Rockland Corporation, 1993, p. 3.

Eisenberg, D. M. "Trends in Alternative Medicine Use in the United States, 1990–1997." *Journal of the American Medical Association,* (Nov. 11, 1998).

Gu, F. "Changes in the Prevalence of Benign Prostatic Hyperplasia in China." *Chinese Medical Journal.* (English version), 1997, 110 (3), 163–166.

Ghaly, F. I. "Energy Medicine: The Wave of the Future." *Healthy and Natural Journal* 6, no. 2 (April 1999): 100–101.

Goldberg, K.A.. et al (editors). *The Complete Book of Men's Health.* Emmaus, Penn.: Rodale Press, 1999.

Heimlich, J. *What Your Doctor Won't Tell You: The Complete Guide to the Latest in Alternative Medicine.* New York: Harper Collins, 1990.

King, D.; J. King; and J. Pearlroth. *Cancer Combat.* New York, N.Y.: Bantam, 1998.

Klausner, R. D. "NIH Consensus Statement." *Acupuncture* 15, no. 5 (Nov 3–5 1997): 19.

Kushi, M. and A. Jack. *The Cancer Prevention Diet.* New York: St. Martin's, 1983.

Leviton, R. "Killing Cancer Cells with Magnetic Energy." *Alternative Medicine Digest* 20 (Oct/Nov 1997): 78–85.

———. "Reversing Cancer Successfully." *Alternative Medicine Digest* 17 (Mar/Apr 1997): 66–69.

Lewis, J. and E. R. Berger. *New Guidelines for Surviving Prostate Cancer.* Westbury, N.Y.: Health Education Literary Publishers, 1997.

Moss, R. W. *Cancer Therapy: The Independent Consumer's Guide to Non-Toxic Treatment and Prevention.* New York: Equinox, 1992.

Murray, M. T. *Natural Alternatives to Over the Counter and Prescription Drugs.* New York: William Morrow, 1994.

Murray, M. T. and J. Pizzorno. *Encyclopedia of Natural Medicine.* Rocklin, Calif.: Prima, 1991.

Preuss, H. G. and B. Adderly. *The Prostate Cure.* New York: Crown, 1998.

Rodriguez, R. and W. C. Moon. *p53 Gene Therapy Program, A Multicenter Prospective, Phase III Study with p53 Gene Therapy in Patients with Advanced Cancer.* San Diego, Calif.: International Health and Education, 1999.

Salmans, S. *Prostate Questions You Have . . . Answers You Need.* Allentown, Penn.: People's Medical Society, 1993.

Siegel, B. S. *Prescriptions for Living.* New York: Harper Collins, 1998.

Simonton, O. C.; S. M. Simonton; and J. Creighton. *Getting Well Again.* Los Angeles: Tarcher, 1978.

Somerville, R. L (project editor). *The Medical Advisor: The Complete Guide to Alternative and Conventional Treatments.* New York: Time Life Books, 1996.

Taub, E. A. *Dr. Taub's 7-Day Program for Radiant Health and Energy.* Englewood Cliffs, N.J.: Prentice Hall, 1994.

Weil, A. *Health and Healing.* Boston: Houghton Mifflin, 1995.

Chapter Six

Adlercreutz, H. et al. "Determination of urinary lignans and phytoestrogen, in urine of women in various habitual diets." *Journal of Steroid Biochemistry* 25 (1986): 791–797.

Atkins, R. C. *Dr. Atkins' Vita Nutrient Solution.* New York: Simon and Schuster, 1998.

Bergman, C. *Modified Citrus Pectin—A Natural Anti-adhesive Agent.* Denmark: Health Form Limited, 1996.

Carraro, J. et al. "Comparison of physiotherapy (Permixon) with Finasteride in the treatment of benign prostate hyperplasia: a randomized international study of 1,098 patients." *Prostate 29* (1996): 231–240.

Clark, L. C.; B. Dalkin; A. Krongrad et al. "Decreased incidence of prostate cancer with selenium supplementation results of a double blind cancer prevention trial." *British Journal of Urology* 81 (1998): 730–734.

Cooper, R. DHA: *The Essential Omega-3 Fatty Acid.* Pleasant Grove, Ut.: Woodland, 1998.

De Silva, D. M. "An angiogenesis primer" *International Journal of Anti-Aging Medicine.* Vol 1, No. 2, Huntington, N.Y., 1998, pp. 14–15.

Giovannucci, E. et al. "Intake of carotenoid and retinol in relation to risk of prostate cancer." *Journal of the National Cancer Institute,* 87:23; 1767–1776.

"Global Nutrition Industry Tops $64 Billion in Sales." *Health Products Business Magazine* (Apr 1999): 10.

"Improved New Form of DHEA, 7-KETO, Replaces DHEA." *Natural Pharmacy News.* Newtown, Penn.: Integrated Health System, vol. 2, no. 3, April 1999, pp. 1–2.

Lau, B. H. S. "Edible plant extracts modulate macrophage activity and bacterial mutagenesis." *International Clinical Nutrition Review.* 12, no. 3 (July 1992): 147–155.

Leake A.; C. D. Chisholm; and F. K. Habib. "The effect of zinc on the 5-alpha-reduction of testosterone by the hyperplasia human prostate gland." *Journal of Steroid Biochemistry,* 20 (1984): 651–655.

Lewis, J. *How I Survived Prostate Cancer . . . and So Can You.* Westbury, N.Y.: Health Education Literary Publishers, 1994.

Lewis, J. and E. R. Berger. *New Guidelines for Surviving Prostate Cancer.* Westbury, N.Y.: Health Education Literary Publishers, 1997.

"Mexican Market for Health Products Grows." *Health Products Business Magazine.* (May 1999): 8.

Milsten, R. and J. Slowinski. *The Sexual Male, Problems and Solutions.* New York: W.W. Norton, 1999, p. 182.

Morgan, B.L.G. and R. Morgan. *Hormones.* Los Angeles: The Body Press, 1989.

Moss, R. W. *Cancer Therapy: The Independent Consumer's Guide to Non-Toxic Treatment and Prevention.* New York: Equinox, 1992.

Murray, M. T. *Natural Alternatives to Over the Counter and Prescription Drugs.* New York: William Morrow, 1994.

"Natural Solutions for a Swollen Prostate." *Alternative Medicine Digest,* 25 (Aug 1998): 14.

Passwater, R. A. *Lipoic Acid: The Metabolic Antioxidant.* New Canaan, Conn.: Keats, 1995.

———."Shark Cartilage and Cancer Revisited, A Follow-up Interview with William Lane." *Whole Food Magazine* 3:95: 60–65.

Pauling, L. and E. Cameron. *Cancer and Vitamin C.* Menlo Park, Calif.: The Linus Pauling Institute of Science and Medicine, 1979.

"PCS." *Alternative Medicine Digest,* 19 (Aug/Sept, 1997): 84–85.

Perlmutter, D. "Good News About Vitamin E." *The Perlmutter Letter* 4, no. 1 (spring 1998): 1.

Pienta, K. et al. "Inhibition of spontaneous metastasis in a rat prostate cancer model by oral administration of modified citrus pectin." *Journal of the National Cancer Institute,* 87 (1995): 348–353.

Poticha, J. and A. Southwood. *Use It or Lose It.* New York: Richard Marek, 1978, p. 85.

Preuss, H. G. and B. Adderly. *The Prostate Cure.* New York: Crown, 1998.

Rogers, S. "How the Sick Get Sicker Quicker Without Nutritional Supplements." *Let's Live* 62, no. 1 (Jan 1994): 44–47.

Shamsuddin, A. M. *IP6: Nature's Revolutionary Cancer Fighter.* New York: Kensington , 1998.

Shealy, C. N. DHEA: *The Youth Hormone.* New Canaan, Conn.: Keats, 1996.

"Soy: Nutritious Food, Powerful Medicine." *Natural Pharmacy News* 2, no. 3 (1999): p. 8.

Weil, A. *Health and Healing.* Boston, Mass.: Houghton Mifflin, 1995.

Weiner, M. A. and J. Weiner. *Herbs That Heal.* Mill Valley, Calif.: Quantum (1994), p. 4.

Whitaker, J. "A Tea That Has Cured Cancer." *Health and Healing, Tomorrow's Medicine Today* 5, no. 5 (1995): p. 4.

Chapter Seven

Airola, P. *How to Get Well.* Phoenix, Ariz.: Health Plus, 1987, p. 24.

Berger, S. *How to Be Your Own Nutritionist.* New York: William Morrow, 1987.

Bland, J. *Assess Your Own Nutritional Status.* New Canaan, Conn.: Keats, 1987.

———. *Medical Applications of Clinical Nutrition.* New Canaan, Conn.: Keats, 1983.

Calbom, C. *Is Nutrition the Missing Piece in the Cancer Treatment Puzzle?* Washington, D.C.: Center for Alternative Cancer Research, 1989.

Cheraskin, E. and W. M. Ringsdorf et al. Diet and Disease. New Canaan, Conn.: Keats, 1987.

Erasmus, U. *Fats That Heal, Fats That Kill.* Menlo Park, Calif.: Designing Health, 1988.

Giovannuci, E. et al. "Intake of carotenoids and retinol in relation to risk of prostate cancer." *Journal of the National Cancer Institute,* 10 (1995): 537–548.

Haas, R. *Permanent Remissions.* New York: Simon and Schuster, 1997.

Kaul, L. et al. "The Role of Diet in Prostate Cancer." *Nutrition and Cancer,* 9 (1987): 123–128.

Keane, M. and D. Chace. *What to Eat if You Have Cancer.* Chicago: Contemporary Books, 1996.

Kervan, L. *Biological Transmutations.* Binghamton, N.Y.: Swan House, 1972.

Landis, R. *Herbal Defense.* New York: Warner, 1997.

Robbins, J. *Diet for a New America.* Walpole, N.H.: Stillpoint, 1987.

Whittemore, A. S. et al. "Prostate cancer in relation to diet, physical activity, and body size in blacks, whites, and Asians in the United States and Canada." *Journal of the National Cancer Institute* 87, no. 9 (May 3, 1995): 652–661.

Chapter Eight

Atkins, R. C. *Dr. Atkins' Vita Nutrient Solution.* New York: Simon and Schuster, 1998.

Cheraskin, E. and W. M. Ringsdorf. *Psycho-Dietetics.* New York: Bantam, 1983, p. 16.

Culp, T. M. "Naturopathic Healing." *Energy Times Magazine* (Jul/Aug 1996): 44–52.

Cummings, S. and D. Ullman. *Everybody's Guide to Homeopathic Medicine.* Los Angeles: Jeremy P. Tarcher, 1984.

De Rosa, G. and S. M. Corsello et al. "Prolactin secretion after beer." *Lancet* 2 (1981): 934.

Dolby, V. "Dr. Atkins: From Diet Guru to Alternative Medicine Champion." *Vitamin Retailer Magazine* (March 1999): 64–66.

Fink, W. *How to Solve the Wellness Puzzle.* Wellesley, Mass.: Burtt, 1986.

Lederman, G. S. *Radioactive Seed Implantation for Prostate Cancer.* (Video). Oncology, New York: State Island University Hospital, Department of Radiation, May 1999.

Masters, W. H.; V. E. Johnson; and R. C. Kolodny. *Crisis: Heterosexual Behavior in the Age of AIDS.* Garden City, N.Y.: Grove, 1988.

Mezzetti, A. et al. "Systemic oxidative stress and its relationship with age and illness." *Journal of American Geriatric Society,* 44 (1996): 823–827.

Morra, M. and E. Potts. *Choices: Realistic Alternatives in Cancer Treatment.* New York: Avon, 1987.

Moss, R. *Cancer Therapy: The Independent Consumer's Guide to Non-Toxic Treatment and Prevention.* New York: Equinox, 1995.

Murray, M. T. and J. E. Pizzorno. *Encyclopedia of Natural Medicine.* Rocklin, Calif.: Prima, 1991.

Pauling, L. *How to Live Longer and Feel Better.* New York: W. H. Freeman, 1986.

Sorge, R. "The Opiates of Optimism." *Visions Magazine,* (Sept 1990): 13.

Starr, C. and R. Taggart. *Biology: The Unity and Diversity of Life.* New York: Wadsworth, 1987.

Walsh, P. C. and J. Farrer. *The Prostate: A Guide for Men and the Women Who Love Them.* Baltimore, Md.: The Johns Hopkins University Press, 1995.

Whitaker, J. T. "Health Lies You've Been Told." *Wellness Today, A Special Supplement to Health and Healing* (Apr 1992): p. 4.

Chapter Nine

Chopra, D. *Quantum Healing.* New York: Bantam, 1989.

Fink, J. *Third Opinion: An International Directory of Alternative Therapy Centers for the Treatment and Prevention of Cancer and Other Degenerative Diseases.* Garden City Park, N.Y.: Avery, 1992.

Lininger, S. "Get Well on Line, A Beginner's Guide to Browsing." *Let's Live Magazine,* 64, no. 10 (Oct 1996): 55–58.

Null, G. "There is Only Individual Transformation." *New Frontier Magazine.* Philadelphia, Penn., vol. xiii, no. 1, Jan./Feb. 1994, pp. 11–12.

Sattilaro, A. J. *Recalled by Life.* Boston: Houghton Mifflin, 1982.

Sorge, R. H. *Nutrition Testing and Personal Evaluation.* Asbury Park, N.J.: Abunda Life, 1981.

Weil, A. *Spontaneous Healing.* New York: Fawcett Columbine, 1995.

INDEX

ABOUT THE AUTHOR

George L. Redmon was born in Edenton, North Carolina and resided most of his life in Philadelphia, Pennsylvania. He graduated with honors and earned his Bachelor's degree in health in 1974. In that same year he was honored as a member of *Who's' Who Among College Students In America.*

Dr. Redmon is a naturopathic physician, a graduate of the Clayton School of Natural Healing, The American Holistic College of Nutrition, and Walden University (1994) where he earned his Ph.D. He has developed a twenty-year career specializing in holistic healthcare. His work has been published in *American Fitness.*

He is a member of the South Jersey Holistic Health Association; the Holistic Health Association of Princeton, New Jersey; the Doctoral Association of New York Educations, Healthier Lifestyles; and the Herbal Healer Academy. Dr. Redmon serves as a consultant to the Center for Stress, Pain and Wellness in Wilmington, Delaware; is on the advisory board of the Clayton School of Natural Health; and teaches as an adjunct faculty member with the Washington Township School system in Sewell, New Jersey. He currently resides in Sicklerville, New Jersey with his wife Brenda, and their son George.

Dr. Redmon is the author of *Minerals: What Your Body Really Needs and Why* (Avery Publishing, 1999), and *Managing and Preventing Arthritis: The Natural Alternatives* (Hohm Press, 1999).

ADDITIONAL HEALTH TITLES FROM HOHM PRESS

10 ESSENTIAL HERBS, REVISED EDITION
by Lalitha Thomas

Peppermint. . .Garlic. . .Ginger. . .Cayenne. . .Clove. . . and 5 other everyday herbs win the author's vote as the "Top 10" most versatile and effective herbal applications for hundreds of health and beauty needs. *Ten Essential Herbs* offers fascinating stories and easy, step-by-step direction for both beginners and seasoned herbalists. Learn how to use cayenne for headaches, how to make a facial scrub with ginger, how to calm motion sickness and other stomach distress with peppermint. Special sections in each chapter explain the application of these herbs with children and pets too. **Over 25,000 copies in print.**

Paper, 395 pages, $16.95   ISBN: 0-934252-48-3

• • •

WRITING YOUR WAY THROUGH CANCER
by Chia Martin

This book applies tried and true methods of journaling and other forms of writing to the particular challenges faced by the cancer patient. Research confirms that people who write about their upsetting experiences show improvement in their immune system functioning. Thousands of cancer patients today could profit from the journal writing techniques and inspiration offered in this practical, comforting, yet non-sentimental, guidebook. Its wisdom is useful to anyone who faces a personal health crisis; or anyone who wishes to confront their grief, loss or a difficult present reality with less panic, fear and confusion.

"Chia Martin's story is a vivid reminder of the importance of psychological and spiritual issues in healthcare." —Larry Dossey, M.D., author, *Reinventing Medicine and Healing Words.*

Paper, 192 pages, $14. 95   ISBN: 1-890772-003

• • •

KAVA: Nature's Relaxant For Anxiety, Stress and Pain
by Hasnain Walji, Ph.D.

KAVA is currently one of the hottest products in the natural medicine and health-food trade. This book provides consumers with a readable introduction and a balanced and authoritative treatment. KAVA has been shown to relieve the anxiety, tension and restlessness that characterize STRESS, a major contributing factor in the most deadly diseases of our times.

Paper, 144 pages, $9.95   ISBN: 0-934252-78-5

TO ORDER PLEASE SEE ACCOMPANYING ORDER FORM OR CALL 1-800-381-2700 TO PLACE YOUR ORDER NOW.

ADDITIONAL HEALTH TITLES FROM HOHM PRESS

YOUR BODY CAN TALK: How to Use Simple Muscle Testing to Listen to What Your Body Knows and Needs
by Susan L. Levy, D.C. and Carol Lehr, M.A.

Clear instructions in **simple muscle testing**, together with over 25 simple tests for how to use it for specific problems or disease conditions. Special chapters deal with health problems specific to women (especially PMS and Menopause) and problems specific to men (like stress, heart disease, and prostate difficulties). Contains over 30 diagrams, plus a complete Index and Resource Guide.

Paper, 350 pages, $19.95   ISBN: 0-934252-68-8

• • •

NATURAL HEALING WITH HERBS
by Humbart "Smokey" Santillo, N.D.
Foreword by Robert S. Mendelsohn, M.D.

Dr. Santillo's first book, and Hohm Press' long-standing bestseller, is a classic handbook on herbal and naturopathic treatment. Acclaimed as the most comprehensive work of its kind, *Natural Healing With Herbs* details (in layperson's terms) the properties and uses of 120 of the most common herbs and lists comprehensive therapies for more than 140 common ailments. All in alphabetical order for quick reference.

 Over 150,000 copies in print.
Paper, 408 pages, $16.95   ISBN: 0-934252-08-4

• • •

10 ESSENTIAL FOODS
by Lalitha Thomas

Carrots, broccoli, almonds, grapefruit and six other miracle foods will enhance your health when used regularly and wisely. Lalitha gives in-depth nutritional information plus flamboyant and good-humored stories about these foods, based on her years of health and nutrition counseling. Each chapter contains easy and delicious recipes, tips for feeding kids and helpful hints for managing your food dollar. A bonus section supports the use of 10 Essential Snacks.

Paper, 300 pages, $16.95   ISBN: 0-934252-74-2

TO ORDER PLEASE SEE ACCOMPANYING ORDER FORM OR CALL 1-800-381-2700 TO PLACE YOUR ORDER NOW.

ADDITIONAL HEALTH TITLES FROM HOHM PRESS

FOOD ENZYMES: THE MISSING LINK TO RADIANT HEALTH
by Humbart "Smokey" Santillo, N.D.

Santillo's breakthrough book presents the most current research in this field, and encourages simple, straightforward steps for how to make enzyme supplementation a natural addition to a nutrition-conscious lifestyle. Special sections on: • Longevity and disease • The value of raw food and juicing • Detoxification • Prevention of allergies and candida • Sports and nutrition

Over 200,000 copies in print.
Paper, 108 pages, U.S. $7.95   ISBN: 0-934252-40-8 (English)
Paper, 108 pages, U.S. $6.95   ISBN: 0-934252-49-1 (Spanish)

■ Audio version of Food Enzymes
2 cassette tapes, 150 minutes, U.S. $17.95   ISBN: 0-934252-29-7

• • •

INTUITIVE EATING: EveryBody's Guide to Vibrant Health and Lifelong Vitality Through Food
by Humbart "Smokey" Santillo, N.D.

The natural voice of the body has been drowned out by the shouts of addictions, over-consumption, and devitalized and preserved foods. Millions battle the scale daily, experimenting with diets and nutritional programs, only to find their victories short-lived at best, confusing and demoralizing at worst. *Intuitive Eating* offers an alternative—a tested method for: • strengthening the immune system • natural weight loss • increasing energy • making the transition from a degenerative diet to a regenerative diet • slowing the aging process.

Paper, 450 pages, $16.95   ISBN: 0-934252-27-0

• • •

THE MELATONIN AND AGING SOURCEBOOK
by Dr. Roman Rozencwaig, M.D. and Dr. Hasnain Walji, Ph.D.

This book covers the latest research on the pineal...control of aging, melatonin and sleep, melatonin and immunity, melatonin's role in cancer treatment, antioxidant qualities of melatonin, dosages, counter indications, quality control, and use with other drugs, melatonin application to heart disease, Alzheimer's, diabetes, stress, major depression, seasonal affective disorders, AIDS, SIDS, cataracts, autism...and many other conditions.

Cloth, 220 pages, $79.95   ISBN: 0-934252-73-4

TO ORDER PLEASE SEE ACCOMPANYING ORDER FORM OR CALL 1-800-381-2700 TO PLACE YOUR ORDER NOW.

ADDITIONAL HEALTH TITLES FROM HOHM PRESS

MANAGING AND PREVENTING ARTHRITIS
The Natural Alternatives
by George L. Redmon, N.D., Ph.D.

Discover a full range of natural alternatives for the prevention of arthritis and other arthritic disturbances, such as gout and fibromyalgia; for slowing the progress of existing arthritis, and for relief of the pain, swelling and stiffness of this disease.

Learn about dietary change as the major form of prevention; the essential role of antioxidants, vitamins and minerals; the use of herbal treatments; revolutionary supplements, such as glucosamaine sulfate; and the irreplaceable role of positive attitude and self-responsibility in managing, treating and preventing arthritis.

Paper, 182 pages, $12.95   ISBN: 0-934252-90-1

• • •

A VEGETARIAN DOCTOR SPEAKS OUT
by Charles Attwood, M.D., F.A.A.P.
By the famed author of *Dr. Attwood's Low-Fat Prescription for Kids* (Viking, 1995), this new book proclaims the life-saving benefits of a plant-based diet. Twenty-six powerful essays speak out against the myths, the prejudices and the ignorance surrounding the subject of nutrition in the U.S. today. Read about the link between high-fat consumption and heart disease, cancer and other killers; the natural and non-dairy way to increase calcium intake; obesity and our children—more than a matter of genes!; controlling food allergies, for the rest of your life, and many more topics of interest and necessity.

Paper, 167 pages, $14.95   ISBN: 0-934252-85-8

• • •

■ *HERBS, NUTRITION AND HEALING ;* AUDIO CASSETTE SERIES
by Dr. Humbart "Smokey" Santillo, N.D.

Santillo's most comprehensive seminar series. Topics covered in-depth include: • the history of herbology • specific preparation of herbs for tinctures, salves, concentrates, etc. • herbal dosages in both acute and chronic illnesses • use of cleansing and transition diets • treating colds and flu... and more.

4 cassettes, 330 minutes, $40.00   ISBN: 0-934252-22-X

TO ORDER PLEASE SEE ACCOMPANYING ORDER FORM OR CALL 1-800-381-2700 TO PLACE YOUR ORDER NOW.

ADDITIONAL HEALTH TITLES FROM HOHM PRESS

■ *NATURE HEALS FROM WITHIN;* AUDIO CASSETTE SERIES
by Dr. Humbart "Smokey" Santillo, N.D.

Topics include: • The innate wisdom of the body. • The essential role of elimination and detoxification • Improving digestion • How "transition dieting" will take off the weight—for good! • The role of heredity, diet, and prevention in health • How to overcome tiredness, improve your immune system and live longer...and happier.

1 cassette, $8.95   ISBN: 0-934252-66-1

• • •

■ *LIVE SEMINAR ON FOOD ENZYMES*; AUDIO CASSETTE SERIES
by Dr. Humbart "Smokey" Santillo, N.D.

An in-depth discussion of the properties of food enzymes, describing their valuable use to maintain vitality, immunity, health and longevity. Complements all the information in the book.

1 cassette, $8.95   ISBN: 0-934252-29-7

• • •

■ *FRUITS AND VEGETABLES—The Basis of Health*; AUDIO CASSETTE SERIES
by Dr. Humbart "Smokey" Santillo, N.D.

Explains the essential difference between a live food diet, which heals the body, and degenerative foods, which weaken the immune system and cause disease. Recipes included.

1 cassette, $8.95   ISBN: 0-934252-65-3

• • •

■ *WEIGHT-LOSS SEMINAR*; AUDIO CASSETTE SERIES
by Dr. Humbart "Smokey" Santillo, N.D.

This seminar explains the worthlessness of most dietary regimens and explodes many common myths about weight gain. Santillo stresses: • The essential distinction between "good" fats and "bad" fats • The necessity for protein and how to use it efficiently • How to get our primary vitamins and minerals from food • How to ease into becoming an "intuitive eater."

1 cassette, $8.95   ISBN: 0-934252-75-0

**TO ORDER PLEASE SEE ACCOMPANYING ORDER FORM
OR CALL 1-800-381-2700 TO PLACE YOUR ORDER NOW.**

ADDITIONAL HEALTH TITLES FROM HOHM PRESS

BEYOND ASPIRIN: Nature's Challenge To Arthritis, Cancer & Alzheimer's Disease
by Thomas A. Newmark and Paul Schulick

A reader-friendly guide to one of the most remarkable medical breakthroughs of our times. Research shows that inhibition of the COX-2 enzyme significantly reduces the inflammation that is currently linked with arthritis, colon and other cancers, and Alzheimer's disease. Challenging the conventional pharmaceutical "silver-bullet" approach, this book pleads a convincing case for the safe and effective use of the COX-2-inhibiting herbs, including green tea, rosemary, basil, ginger, turmeric and others.

Paper, 340 pages, $14.95   ISBN: 0-934252-82-3
Cloth, 340 pages, $24.95   ISBN: 1-890772-01-1

• • •

MANAGING AND PREVENTING PROSTATE DISORDERS
The Natural Alternatives
by George L. Redmon, N.D., Ph.D.

Well-established and current research indicates that prostate disorders are largely preventable, and for those already afflicted its symptoms are manageable by a wide variety of natural means. This book about prostate health contains lifesaving information that every man, and his family, should know about:

· Who is at Risk?
· Prevention Options
· Safe, Natural Treatments for Prostate Disorders including * nutrition and dietary recommendations * enzyme therapies * energy medicine * highly effective herbs and supplements *detoxification programs and more.

Contains a complete Resource and Referral Guide

Paper, 220 pages, $12.95   ISBN: 0-934252-97-1

TO ORDER PLEASE SEE ACCOMPANYING ORDER FORM OR CALL 1-800-381-2700 TO PLACE YOUR ORDER NOW.

RETAIL ORDER FORM FOR HOHM PRESS HEALTH BOOKS

Name_____ Phone (   ) _____

Street Address or P.O. Box _____

City _____ State _____ Zip Code _____

	QTY	TITLE	ITEM PRICE	TOTAL PRICE
1		**10 ESSENTIAL FOODS**	$16.95	
2		**10 ESSENTIAL HERBS**	$16.95	
3		**MANAGING AND PREVENTING ARTHRITIS**	$12.95	
4		**BEYOND ASPIRIN** Paper	$14.95	
5		**BEYOND ASPIRIN** Cloth	$24.95	
6		**WRITING YOUR WAY THROUGH CANCER**	$14.95	
7		**FOOD ENZYMES/ENGLISH**	$7.95	
8		**FOOD ENZYMES/SPANISH**	$6.95	
9		**FOOD ENZYMES BOOK/AUDIO**	$17.95	
10		**FRUITS & VEGETABLES/AUDIO**	$8.95	
11		**HERBS, NUTRITION AND HEALING/AUDIO**	$40.00	
12		**INTUITIVE EATING**	$16.95	
13		**LIVE SEMINAR ON FOOD ENZYMES/AUDIO**	$8.95	
14		**MANAGING & PREVENTING PROSTATE DISORD.**	$12.95	
15		**THE MELATONIN AND AGING SOURCEBOOK**	$79.95	
16		**NATURAL HEALING WITH HERBS**	$16.95	
17		**NATURE HEALS FROM WITHIN/AUDIO**	$8.95	
18		**A VEGETARIAN DOCTOR SPEAKS OUT**	$14.95	
19		**WEIGHT LOSS SEMINAR/AUDIO**	$8.95	
20		**YOUR BODY CAN TALK: How to Listen...**	$19.95	

SURFACE SHIPPING CHARGES

1st book $5.00
Each additional item $1.00

SUBTOTAL:
SHIPPING: (see below)
TOTAL:

SHIP MY ORDER

☐ Surface U.S. Mail—Priority   ☐ UPS (Mail + $2.00)
☐ 2nd-Day Air (Mail + $5.00)   ☐ Next-Day Air (Mail + $15.00)

METHOD OF PAYMENT:

☐ Check or M.O.   Payable to Hohm Press, P.O. Box 2501, Prescott, AZ 86302
☐ Call 1-800-381-2700 to place your credit card order
☐ Or call 1-520-717-1779 to fax your credit card order
☐ Information for Visa/MasterCard order only:

Card #_____ – _____ – _____ – _____   Expiration Date _____

Visit our Website to view our complete catalog: www.hohmpress.com
ORDER NOW! Call 1-800-381-2700 or fax your order to 1-520-717-1779.
(Remember to include your credit card information.)

RETAIL ORDER FORM FOR HOHM PRESS HEALTH BOOKS

Name_____ Phone (_____) _____

Street Address or P.O. Box _____

City _____ State _____ Zip Code _____

	QTY	TITLE	ITEM PRICE	TOTAL PRICE
1		**10 ESSENTIAL FOODS**	$16.95	
2		**10 ESSENTIAL HERBS**	$16.95	
3		**MANAGING AND PREVENTING ARTHRITIS**	$12.95	
4		**BEYOND ASPIRIN** Paper	$14.95	
5		**BEYOND ASPIRIN** Cloth	$24.95	
6		**WRITING YOUR WAY THROUGH CANCER**	$14.95	
7		**FOOD ENZYMES/ENGLISH**	$7.95	
8		**FOOD ENZYMES/SPANISH**	$6.95	
9		**FOOD ENZYMES BOOK/AUDIO**	$17.95	
10		**FRUITS & VEGETABLES/AUDIO**	$8.95	
11		**HERBS, NUTRITION AND HEALING/AUDIO**	$40.00	
12		**INTUITIVE EATING**	$16.95	
13		**LIVE SEMINAR ON FOOD ENZYMES/AUDIO**	$8.95	
14		**MANAGING & PREVENTING PROSTATE DISORD.**	$12.95	
15		**THE MELATONIN AND AGING SOURCEBOOK**	$79.95	
16		**NATURAL HEALING WITH HERBS**	$16.95	
17		**NATURE HEALS FROM WITHIN/AUDIO**	$8.95	
18		**A VEGETARIAN DOCTOR SPEAKS OUT**	$14.95	
19		**WEIGHT LOSS SEMINAR/AUDIO**	$8.95	
20		**YOUR BODY CAN TALK: How to Listen...**	$19.95	

SURFACE SHIPPING CHARGES

1st book $5.00

Each additional item $1.00

SUBTOTAL: _____

SHIPPING: (see below) _____

TOTAL: _____

SHIP MY ORDER

☐ Surface U.S. Mail—Priority   ☐ UPS (Mail + $2.00)

☐ 2nd-Day Air (Mail + $5.00)   ☐ Next-Day Air (Mail + $15.00)

METHOD OF PAYMENT:

☐ Check or M.O.   Payable to Hohm Press, P.O. Box 2501, Prescott, AZ 86302

☐ Call 1-800-381-2700 to place your credit card order

☐ Or call 1-520-717-1779 to fax your credit card order

☐ Information for Visa/MasterCard order only:

Card #_____ – _____ – _____ – _____   Expiration Date _____

Visit our Website to view our complete catalog: www.hohmpress.com

ORDER NOW! Call 1-800-381-2700 or fax your order to 1-520-717-1779.

(Remember to include your credit card information.)